Macleod's Essentials of Examination

Macleod's Essentials of Examination

Euan A Sandilands
MD FRCP(Edin) PGCert (MedEd)
Consultant Physician,
Clinical Toxicology and Acute Medicine,
National Poisons Information Service,
Royal Infirmary of Edinburgh, Edinburgh, UK

Katharine Strachan
MA FRCP(Edin)
Consultant Physician,
Acute and General Medicine,
Clinical Lead Medical Ethics Education,
Royal Infirmary of Edinburgh, Edinburgh, UK

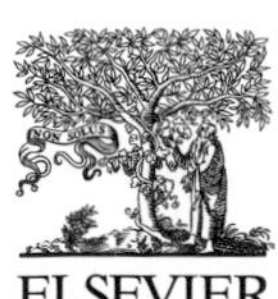

ELSEVIER Edinburgh London New York Oxford Philadelphia St Louis Sydney 2020

Elsevier

Notices

Practitioners and researchers must always rely on their own experience and knowledge in evaluating and using any information, methods, compounds or experiments described herein. Because of rapid advances in the medical sciences, in particular, independent verification of diagnoses and drug dosages should be made. To the fullest extent of the law, no responsibility is assumed by Elsevier, authors, editors or contributors for any injury and/or damage to persons or property as a matter of products liability, negligence or otherwise, or from any use or operation of any methods, products, instructions, or ideas contained in the material herein.

ISBN: 978-0-7020-7872-9

Executive Content Strategist: Laurence Hunter
Content Development Specialist: Carole McMurray
Content Coordinator: Susan Jansons
Project Manager: Anne Collett
Design: Miles Hitchen
Marketing Manager: Deborah Watkins

Printed in China

Last digit is the print number: 9 8 7 6 5 4 3 2 1

Contents

Preface

Innovations in technology have enhanced the diagnostic capabilities of today's practising clinicians. However, the traditional art of detecting clinical signs through expert examination techniques still remains a fundamental competence for training and practising clinicians, central to the delivery of safe and effective patient care. In this first edition of *Macleod's Essential Examination,* we have provided a concise account of each system examination, delivering the information in a compact and portable format for use at home and in the clinical environment. A basic level of knowledge and understanding of examination technique is assumed and it is intended therefore that this book is read in conjunction with *Macleod's Clinical Examination* with which it is closely integrated.

How to use this book

This book is intended to be a practical aide-memoire of each system-based examination that will assist in preparation for OSCEs and clinical practice. Each chapter follows the same format, opening with typical OSCE scenarios followed by a concise 'point by point' examination template. Over the following pages, the examination template is repeated and expanded with a detailed description of each aspect of the examination process including specific instructions around technique and information about clinical signs to consider. Additionally, exam tips are provided, including typical questions you may be asked during an OSCE. Answers to these questions are displayed at the end of each chapter, allowing the book to be used as a self-assessment tool or in peer-to-peer learning.

1

The cardiovascular system

Common OSCE openers

1. Please examine the cardiovascular system
2. This patient has breathlessness/chest pain/palpitations; please examine them
3. Please examine the precordium (in this scenario omit points 5–7 & 14)

The cardiovascular exam: point by point

1. Introduction
2. Inspection
3. Hands
4. Pulse
5. Face
6. Eyes/Mouth
7. Jugular venous pressure (JVP)
8. Precordium
9. Apex beat
10. Heaves/Thrills
11. Auscultate
12. Manoeuvres ×2
13. Lung bases/Sacral oedema
14. Ankles
15. Conclusion

	The cardiovascular exam: point by point in action		
	DO	**THINK!**	**EXAM TIPS**
1	• Wash hands, introduce yourself • Confirm name/DOB • Position patient at 45°	• Ensure patient adequately exposed • Maintain dignity	• Be professional • Use your full name
2	• Inspect from end of bed (10 seconds)	• Comfortable, breathless, in pain? • Oxygen, medication, observation chart?	• Count to 10 in your head as you inspect from the end of the bed. It calms your nerves before you start examining.
3	• Inspect hands and nails • Feel temperature • Check capillary refill (normal <2 secs)	• Peripheral cyanosis: peripheral vascular disease (PVD), Raynaud's phenomenon • Skin crease pallor: anaemia • Tendon xanthomata: hypercholesterolaemia • Osler's nodes/Janeway lesions: infective endocarditis (IE) • Finger clubbing: IE, cyanotic congenital heart disease • Koilonychia/leuconychia: iron/albumin deficiency • Splinter haemorrhages: IE, trauma • Nailfold infarcts: vasculitis, systemic lupus erythematosus (SLE)	• Lots to think about but very quick part of examination – don't spend longer than than 30 secs • For the causes of finger clubbing see page 17 **Q1** What are the peripheral stigmata of IE?
4	• Time radial pulse (15 secs) • Palpate both radial pulses simultaneously checking for delay • Check collapsing pulse (radial) • Check carotid pulse (warn patient)	• Rate/rhythm/volume/character • Collapsing pulse: aortic regurgitation (AR) • Slow rising pulse: aortic stenosis (AS)	• Ensure heart rate you report is divisible by 4 **Q2** Describe common pulse abnormalities **Q3** What are the common causes of atrial fibrillation?
5	• Inspect face	• Malar flush: mitral stenosis (MS)	
6	• Pull down lower eyelid and check conjunctivae • Look on underside of tongue	• Corneal arcus/xanthelasma: hypercholesterolaemia • Central cyanosis: congenital heart disease, right heart failure	• Xanthelasma and corneal arcus also occur in normolipidaemic patients • Xanthelasma is an independent risk factor for coronary heart disease; corneal arcus has no prognostic value

The cardiovascular exam: point by point in action

	DO	THINK!	EXAM TIPS
7	• Examine JVP • Check hepatojugular reflex	• JVP reflects right atrial pressure • Hepatojugular reflex represents distension of neck veins when pressure is applied over the liver	• Assessed by observing level of pulsation in the internal jugular vein (not external, which is easier to see) with patient at 45 degrees • Normal: <4 cm above sternal angle **Q4a** Describe the waveforms of the JVP **Q4b** Describe the abnormalities of the JVP
8	• Expose precordium	• Midline sternotomy scar: coronary artery bypass graft (CABG)/valve replacement (if scar present, look at legs for venous grafting scar) • Left submammary scar: mitral valvotomy or transapical transcatheter aortic valve implantation • Infraclavicular scar (R or L): pacemaker/implantable cardioverter defibrillator (ICD)	• Pacemaker/ICD often missed under clothing – expose and feel for mass
9	• Apex beat	• Impalpable: obesity, asthma, emphysema • Displaced: left ventricular (LV) dilatation (e.g. post myocardial infarction [MI]), severe AR, decompensated AS, dilated cardiomyopathy • Undisplaced thrusting: left ventricular hypertrophy (LVH) (e.g. hypertension, AS) • Undisplaced tapping apex beat (palpable first heart sound): MS • Double apical impulse: hypertrophic cardiomyopathy	• The apex beat should be palpable in the 5th intercostal space and midclavicular line • If palpable, physically count out rib spaces to locate apex • If you cannot feel the apex beat, ask patient to roll on to their left side

The cardiovascular exam: point by point in action

	DO	THINK!	EXAM TIPS
10	• Palpate for heaves and thrills	• Left parasternal heave: right ventricular hypertrophy (RVH) • Most common thrill: AS palpable over the upper right sternal border	• Heave: palpable impulse lifting your hand. Ask patient to hold their breath in expiration. • Thrill: tactile equivalent of murmur
11	• Auscultate	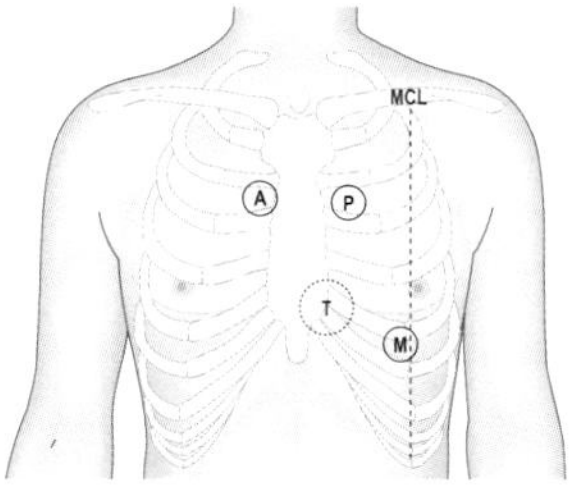 **Fig. 1.1 Sites for auscultation.** Sites at which murmurs from the relevant valves arc usually, but not preferentially, heard. • Systolic murmur radiating to axilla: mitral regurgitation (MR) • Systolic murmur radiating to carotids: AS	• Know difference between the bell and the diaphragm • Listen in each area once in order • Palpate carotid while auscultating • Listen over the carotid arteries for radiation (AS) or carotid bruits
12	• Manoeuvres accentuate diastolic murmurs • Roll patient on to their left hand side, ask them to hold their breath in expiration and listen with the bell at the apex • Sit patient up, ask them to hold their breath in expiration and listen with the diaphragm at the lower left sternal edge	• Diastolic murmur at apex on left hand side: MS • Diastolic murmur at lower left sternal edgc sitting up: AR	• Inspiration amplifies right-sided murmurs • Expiration amplifies left-sided murmurs **Q5** Identify the murmur **Q6** Define the grades of murmurs
13	• Auscultate lung bases • Palpate for sacral oedema	• Crepitations at lung bases: pulmonary oedema • Sacral oedema: right heart failure (RHF), congestive cardiac failure	• Perform immediately after sitting patient up for AR manoeuvre
14	• Palpate ankles	• Peripheral oedema: RHF, congestive cardiac failure	**Q7** What are the causes of peripheral oedema?

The cardiovascular exam: point by point in action			
	DO	THINK!	EXAM TIPS
15	• To complete my exam I would check the blood pressure (BP), peripheral pulses and request a urinalysis (blood: IE) • Thank patient • Wash hands	• Always finish with a concluding statement to clearly indicate completion of the exam	Q8 What is the definition of hypertension? Q9 Describe the treatment of hypertension

Classic OSCE questions

Q1 Peripheral stigmata of IE	
Hands	Janeway lesions Osler nodes
Nails	Splinter haemorrhages
Eyes	Roth spots (fundoscopy) Petechial haemorrhages on conjunctivae

Notes

Q2 Pulse abnormalities

Abnormality	Sinus rhythm	Arrhythmia
Fast rate (tachycardia, >100 bpm)	Exercise Pain Excitement/anxiety Fever Hyperthyroidism Medication: Sympathomimetics, e.g. salbutamol, vasodilators	Atrial fibrillation Atrial flutter Supraventricular tachycardia Ventricular tachycardia
Slow rate (bradycardia, <60 bpm)	Sleep Athletic training Hypothyroidism Medication: Beta-blockers, digoxin	Carotid sinus hypersensitivity Sick sinus syndrome Second-degree heart block Complete heart block
Irregular pulse	Sinus arrhythmia Atrial extrasystoles Ventricular extrasystoles	Atrial fibrillation Atrial flutter with variable response Second-degree heart block with variable response

Notes

Q3 Causes of atrial fibrillation

Hypertension Heart failure Myocardial infarction Thyrotoxicosis Alcohol-related heart disease	Mitral valve disease Infection, e.g. respiratory, urinary Following surgery, especially cardiothoracic surgery

Q4a Waveforms of the JVP

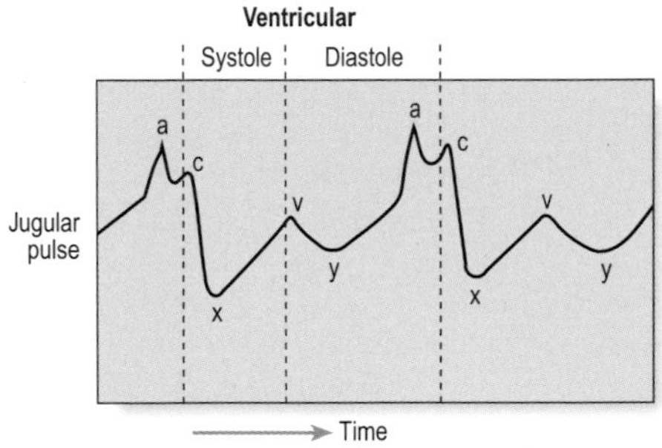

Ventricular
Systole
Diastole
Jugular pulse
a
c
v
x
y
Time

Fig. 1.2 Jugular venous pressure. Form of the venous pulse wave tracing from the internal jugular vein: a, atrial systole; c, closure of the tricuspid valve; v, peak pressure in right atrium immediately prior to opening of tricuspid valve; a–x, descent, due to downward displacement of the tricuspid ring during systole; v–y, descent at commencement of ventricular filling.

Q4b Abnormalities of the JVP

Heart failure	Elevated
PE	Elevated
Pericardial effusion	Elevated, prominent y descent
Pericardial constriction	Elevated, Kussmaul's sign (rises with inspiration, falls with expiration)
Superior vena cava (SVC) obstruction	Elevated, loss of pulsation
Atrial fibrillation (AF)	Absent 'a' waves
Tricuspid stenosis	Giant 'a' waves
Tricuspid regurgitation	Giant 'v' waves
Complete heart block	'Cannon' waves

Notes

Q5a Common causes of a systolic murmur

	Aortic stenosis	Mitral regurgitation
Type	Ejection systolic murmur	Pan-systolic murmur
Causes	Rheumatic heart disease Calcified congenital bicuspid valve (presenting in middle age) Calcified normal tricuspid valve (presenting in elderly)	Rheumatic heart disease Infective endocarditis Mitral valve prolapse Papillary muscle rupture (post MI) 'Functional' MR secondary to left ventricular (LV) dilatation Hypertrophic cardiomyopathy Marfan's syndrome SLE Ehlers–Danlos syndrome
Symptoms	Syncope Dyspnoea Angina	Dyspnoea Heart failure
Investigations	ECG: LVH/LV strain CXR: normal heart size Echo: Doppler examination to assess pressure gradient across valve	ECG: AF common CXR: Cardiomegaly, pulmonary oedema Echo: Doppler and colour flow Doppler used to measure severity
Medical management	Treat hypertension	Treat AF, heart failure (diuretics, angiotensin-converting enzyme inhibitors [ACEi]) Anticoagulation
Indications for surgery	Severe disease plus symptoms or LV impairment Moderate/severe disease and undergoing CABG Some recommend surgery for asymptomatic patients with critical aortic stenosis (valve area <0.6 cm^2 or valve gradient >50 mmHg) Transcatheter aortic valve implantation (TAVI) may be considered if unfit for open surgery	Symptomatic patients with severe disease or LV impairment Asymptomatic patients with severe MR and preserved LV function may be considered for surgery in presence of AF and/or pulmonary hypertension Emergency valve replacement for acute severe MR

Notes

Q5b Common causes of a diastolic murmur

	Aortic regurgitation	Mitral stenosis
Type	Blowing early diastolic murmur at left sternal edge	Mid-diastolic murmur after a loud first heart sound and opening snap
Causes	Rheumatic heart disease Infective endocarditis* Bicuspid aortic valve Aortic dissection* Marfan's syndrome Rheumatoid arthritis Ankylosing spondylitis **cause of acute aortic regurgitation*	Rheumatic heart disease
Symptoms	Dyspnoea Palpitations	Dyspnoea Pulmonary oedema Cough productive of blood tinged sputum Pulmonary hypertension leads to RHF
Investigations	CXR: Cardiomegaly, pulmonary oedema ECG: LV hypertrophy Echo: Doppler examination to assess severity	ECG: AF common, P mitrale CXR: Enlarged left atrium Echo: valve area <2 cm^2 moderate MS, <1 cm^2 severe
Medical management	Diuretics, vasodilators	Treat AF, heart failure (diuretics, ACEi) Anticoagulation
Indications for surgery	Severe disease plus symptoms or LV impairment Surgery should not be delayed until there is irreversible LV dysfunction	Moderate/severe disease Percutaneous balloon valvuloplasty preferred Open repair/replacement if persistent LA thrombus, rigid calcified valve

Notes

Q6 Grades of intensity of murmur

Grade	Description
1	Heard by an expert in optimum conditions
2	Heard by a non-expert in optimum conditions
3	Easily heard; no thrill
4	A loud murmur, with a thrill
5	Very loud, often heard over a wide area, with thrill
6	Extremely loud, heard without a stethoscope

Q7 Causes of peripheral oedema

Unilateral	Deep vein thrombosis (DVT) Trauma Soft-tissue infection Lymphoedema
Bilateral	Heart fure Chronic venous insufficiency Hypoproteinaemia, e.g. nephrotic syndrome, cirrhosis Drugs (nonsteroidal anti-inflammatory drugs [NSAIDs], amlodipine) Inferior vena cava (IVC) obstructionail

Notes

Q8 Definition of hypertension

Stage 1	Clinic >140/90 and daytime ABPM >135/85
Stage 2	Clinic >160/100 and daytime ABPM >150/95
Severe	Clinic SBP >180 or DBP >110

ABPM, ambulatory blood pressure monitoring; DBP, diastolic blood pressure; SBP, systolic blood pressure.
Reproduced from the National Institute for Health and Care Excellence (NICE) guidelines www.nice.org.uk.

Q9 Treatment of hypertension

	Age <55 years*	Age >55 years or black African/Caribbean origin
Step 1	ACEi or ARB	CCB
Step 2	ACEi or ARB + CCB or thiazide diuretic	CCB + ACEi or ARB or thiazide diuretic
Step 3	ACEi or ARB + CCB + thiazide diuretic	CCB + ACEi or ARB + thiazide diuretic
Step 4	Resistant hypertension Options include spironolactone, alpha blocker, beta blocker Seek specialist advice	Resistant hypertension Options include spironolactone, alpha blocker, beta blocker Seek specialist advice

*If the patient has hypertension and type 2 diabetes then treat according to this column.
ACEi, angiotensin converting enzyme inhibitor; ARB, angiotensin receptor blocker; CCB, calcium channel blocker. Reproduced from the National Institute for Health and Care Excellence (NICE) guidelines www.nice.org.uk.

Notes

2

The respiratory system

Common OSCE openers

1. Please examine the respiratory system
2. This patient is breathless/has a cough/has chest pain; please examine them
3. Please examine the chest (in this scenario omit points 3–8)

The respiratory exam: point by point

1. Introduction
2. Inspection
3. Hands
4. Asterixis (flapping tremor)
5. Face/Eyes/Mouth
6. Trachea
7. Jugular venous pressure (JVP)
8. Lymph nodes
9. Inspection from the back
10. Palpation
11. Percussion
12. Auscultation
13. Vocal resonance
14. Repeat 9–13 from the front
15. Conclusion

The respiratory exam: point by point in action

	DO	THINK!	EXAM TIPS
1	• Wash hands, introduce yourself • Confirm name/DOB • Position patient at 45°	• Ensure patient adequately exposed • Maintain dignity	• Be professional • Use your full name
2	• Inspect from end of bed (10 seconds)	• Comfortable, breathless, cyanosed? • Chest shape, accessory muscle use, pursed lip breathing? • Oxygen, medication, observation chart? • Peak flow, sputum pot, nebulisers?	• Count to 10 in your head as you inspect from the end of the bed. It calms your nerves before you start examining. • Look inside a sputum pot!
3	• Inspect hands and nails • Feel temperature • Check pulse (15 seconds) and respiratory rate (15 seconds)	• Tar (**not** nicotine) staining: smoking • Temperature: central cyanosis (warm) vs peripheral cyanosis (cold) • Peripheral cyanosis: peripheral vascular disease (PVD), Raynaud's • Finger clubbing • Small muscle wasting: T1 root damage by apical lung tumour • Yellow nail syndrome: lymphoedema and exudative pleural effusion	• Lots to think about but this should be a quick part of the examination. Don't spend longer than 30 seconds on this. **Q1** What are the causes of finger clubbing?
4	• Asterixis (flapping tremor)	• Fine tremor: β_2 agonist treatment • Coarse flapping tremor: CO_2 retention, hepatic encephalopathy • Unilateral: structural abnormality of contralateral hemisphere	• Flapping tremor is caused by intermittent failure of parietal mechanisms to maintain posture
5	• Inspect face • Pull lower eyelid down and check conjunctivae • Look on underside of tongue	• Cushingoid appearance: long term steroid use • Swelling of face/neck/trunk: superior vena cava obstruction (SVC) (skin usually dusky in appearance) • Conjunctival pallor: anaemia • Horner's syndrome • Central cyanosis: hypoxia, cardiac shunt • Candida: steroid inhalers, immunocompromised	**Q2** What are the side effects of long term corticosteroids? **Q3** What are the features of Horner's syndrome? **Q4** What causes Horner's syndrome?

The respiratory exam: point by point in action

	DO	THINK!	EXAM TIPS
6	• Palpate trachea (warn patient) • Check cricosternal distance (normal is 3–4 fingers)	• Cricosternal distance reduced: chronic obstructive pulmonary disease (COPD) • Is the trachea central or deviated to one side?	**Q5** What are the common causes of tracheal deviation?
7	• Examine the JVP	• See page 7 for abnormalities of the JVP	**Q6** What are the clinical signs and causes of SVC obstruction?
8	**Sit patient forward** • Examine lymph nodes	• Check if painful first • Palpate symmetrically • Tender: infection • Non-tender: possibly malignant	• Palpable nodes fixed to deep structures or skin are usually malignant
9	**From the back** • Inspect the chest	• AP diameter should be < lateral • AP > lateral (barrel chest): COPD • Pectus excavatum (funnel chest): developmental deformity • Pectus carinatum (pigeon chest): prominence of sternum • (Kypho)scoliosis • Scars: lobectomy, pneumonectomy	• Always take time to check for scars which are easy to miss when nervous in the exam setting
10	• Palpation • Assess chest expansion • When examining from front (see point 14) also check apex beat	• Reduced expansion indicates pathology on that side (effusion, collapse, pneumothorax) • Bilateral reduction in chest expansion: severe COPD, fibrosis • Displaced apex beat: mediastinal shift caused by collapse, tension pneumothorax, large pleural effusion • Impalpable apex beat: hyperinflation in COPD causes the lingula of left upper lobe to come between heart and chest wall • Right ventricular heave: pulmonary hypertension	• Assess chest expansion on the upper and lower chest wall • Asymmetry is more important than the degree of expansion • Ribs normally move out and up with inspiration • In COPD the normal outward movement of the lower ribs on inspiration is replaced by paradoxical inward movement due to abnormally low flat diaphragm (Hoover's sign)

The respiratory exam: point by point in action

	DO	THINK!	EXAM TIPS
11	• Percussion • Start in supraclavicular fossae and work down, comparing side to side	• Resonant, dull, stony dull, hyper-resonant	• Ask patient to sit forward with arms folded in front to move the scapulae laterally **Q7** What are the causes of percussion note abnormalities?
12	• Auscultation	• Are the breath sounds vesicular or bronchial? • Wheeze, crepitations • Pleural rub	• Use the same sequence of sites as percussion • Normal secretions clear with coughing **Q8** What are the causes of bronchial breathing?
13	• Vocal resonance	• '1-1-1' or '99' • Increased: consolidation • Decreased: collapse/effusion/ pneumothorax • Ask the patient to whisper and repeat	• Whispering is not heard over normal lung, but sound is transmitted across a consolidated lung: whispering pectoriloquy
14	• Repeat 9–13 from front		• Most information is gained from the back. The examiner may stop you here but always announce your intention to examine from the front
15	• To complete my exam I would check the oxygen saturations and peak flow.	• Always finish with a concluding statement to clearly indicate completion of the exam	**Q9** What are the causes of acid/base abnormalities?

Classic OSCE questions

Q1 Causes of finger clubbing

Congenital or familial	
Respiratory	Lung cancer Bronchiectasis Lung abscess Empyema Cystic fibrosis
Cardiovascular	Cyanotic congenital heart disease Infective endocarditis Arteriovenous (AV) shunts
Gastrointestinal	Cirrhosis Inflammatory bowel disease (IBD) Coeliac disease
Others	Thyrotoxicosis

Q2 Side effects of corticosteroids

Skin	Acne Atrophy Purpura
Cardiovascular	Hypertension
Endocrine	Weight gain Hyperglycaemia Osteoporosis Adrenal insufficiency
Eyes	Cataract Glaucoma
Central nervous system (CNS)	Psychosis
Gastrointestinal	Peptic ulceration
Other	Immunosuppression Avascular bone necrosis

Notes

Q3 Horner's syndrome

Group of symptoms caused by damage to sympathetic trunk	
Symptoms occur on same side as lesion	
Features	Miosis Partial ptosis Anhidrosis Enophthalmos

Q4 Causes of Horner's syndrome

Central	Syringomyelia Multiple sclerosis (MS) Encephalitis Brain tumour
Preganglionic	Pancoast tumour Thyroid cancer Thyroidectomy Goitre Cervical rib
Postganglionic	Carotid artery dissection Cavernous sinus thrombosis Migraine Cluster headache (Horton's headache)

Q5 Tracheal deviation

Towards lung lesion	Upper lobe or lung collapse Upper lobe fibrosis Pneumonectomy
Away from lung lesion	Tension pneumothorax Pleural effusion
Other	Retrosternal goitre Lymphoma Lung cancer

Notes

Q6 SVC obstruction	
Features	Non-pulsatile elevated JVP Abdominojugular reflex absent Facial flushing Distension of neck veins Stridor when arms above head
Causes	Lung cancer Lymphoma Thymoma Mediastinal fibrosis

Q7 Percussion note	
Resonant	Normal
Hyperresonant	Pneumothorax
Dull	Consolidation Collapse Severe pulmonary fibrosis
Stony dull	Pleural effusion Haemothorax

Q8 Causes of bronchial breathing	
Common	Consolidation
Uncommon	Localised pulmonary fibrosis At the top of a pleural effusion Collapsed lung (where bronchus still patent)

Notes

Q9a Causes of respiratory acidosis/alkalosis

	Respiratory acidosis	Respiratory alkalosis
pH	↓	↑
H^+	↑	↓
CO_2	↑	↓
HCO_3	↑ (compensated)	↓ (compensated)
Causes	Severe acute asthma Severe pneumonia Exacerbation COPD Thoracic skeletal abnormality (kyphoscoliosis) Neuromuscular (e.g. muscular dystrophy) CNS depression: • Drug induced e.g. opiates, benzodiazepines • Head trauma • Post-ictal states	Pregnancy High altitude Hyperventilation (anxiety, panic) CNS causes (e.g. stroke, subarachnoid haemorrhage [SAH]) Salicylate poisoning

Q9b Causes of metabolic acidosis/alkalosis

	Metabolic acidosis	Metabolic alkalosis
pH	↓	↑
H^+	↑	↓
CO_2	↓ (compensated)	↑ (compensated)
HCO_3	↓	↑
Causes	Increased production of acid: • Diabetic ketoacidosis • Poisoning (e.g. alcohol, iron, salicylate, methanol, ethylene glycol) • Lactic acidosis (e.g. shock) Loss of bicarbonate: • Renal tubular acidosis • Diarrhoea • Addison's disease	Gastrointestinal acid loss: • Severe vomiting Renal acid loss: • Primary hyperaldosteronism (Conn syndrome) • Secondary hyperaldosteronism: e.g. volume depletion (diuretics), heart failure, Cushing syndrome • Hypokalaemia commonly occurs in above states and perpetuates metabolic alkalosis

3

The abdominal system

Common OSCE openers

1. Please examine the gastrointestinal system
2. This patient presents with weight loss and abdominal pain; please examine them
3. This patient presents with jaundice; please examine their abdomen

The abdominal exam: point by point

1. Introduction
2. Inspection
3. Hands
4. Face/Eyes
5. Mouth
6. Neck
7. Inspect/palpate abdomen
8. Palpate liver
9. Palpate spleen
10. Palpate kidneys
11. Shifting dullness
12. Auscultate
13. Legs
14. Conclusion

The abdominal exam: point by point in action

	DO	THINK!	EXAM TIPS
1	• Wash hands, introduce yourself • Confirm name/DOB • Position patient at 45°	• Ensure patient adequately exposed • Maintain dignity	• Be professional • Use your full name
2	• Inspect from end of bed (10 seconds)	• Comfortable, in pain, cachectic, well nourished? • Loss of body hair/spider naevi: chronic liver disease (CLD) • Gynaecomastia: drugs (spironolactone, digoxin), CLD (see page 96) • Bruising: CLD (thrombocytopenia, reduced synthesis of clotting factors) • Intravenous drug use (IVDU) marks/tattoos: risks for viral hepatitis	• Count to 10 in your head as you inspect from the end of the bed. It calms your nerves before you start examining.
3	• Inspect hands and nails • Check for asterixis (flapping tremor)	• Finger clubbing (see page 17) • Palmar erythema: CLD, pregnancy, hyperthyroidism, rheumatoid arthritis (RA) • Leuconychia (white nails): CLD, other hypoalbuminaemic states • Koilonychia (spoon-shaped nails): iron deficiency • Dupuytren's contracture (feel palm): alcohol-related liver disease, diabetes, trauma, familial • Asterixis: liver failure (encephalopathy)	• Lots to think about but very quick part of examination – no more than 30 seconds **Q1** What are the peripheral stigmata of CLD?
4	• Inspect face for parotid swelling • Pull down lower eyelid and check conjunctivae	• Parotid swelling: chronic alcohol misuse • Icteric sclera: hyperbilirubinaemia • Conjunctival pallor: iron deficiency • Episcleritis/conjunctivitis: inflammatory bowel disease (IBD)	**Q2** What are the common causes of jaundice?

The abdominal exam: point by point in action

	DO	THINK!	EXAM TIPS
5	• Inspect mouth and tongue	• Angular cheilitis/atrophic glossitis: iron deficiency • Beefy/raw tongue: B_{12}/folate deficiency • Mouth ulcers: IBD • Oral candidiasis: immunodeficiency • Fetor hepaticus (musty/sweet breath): liver failure	
6	• Palpate neck for lymphadenopathy	• Troisier's sign: enlarged left supraclavicular Virchow's node; considered a sign of metastatic abdominal malignancy	• Widespread lymphadenopathy may indicate lymphoma (check for hepatosplenomegaly)
7	• Position patient supine with head resting on 1–2 pillows only • Expose abdomen from xiphisternum to symphysis pubis • Ask patient whether they have abdominal pain. If so, where? • Palpate for tenderness/masses	• Abdominal striae: weight gain e.g., Cushing's syndrome • Loose skin folds: weight loss • Distension: everted umbilicus • Recent ascitic drain scar • Caput medusae: portal hypertension • Scars/stomas (Fig. 3.1) • Note any palpable mass (Fig. 3.2)	• Ensure you are at level of bed when palpating abdomen and watch patient's face throughout • Start away from any area of tenderness **Q3** Identify the abdominal scar **Q4** Describe the different surgical stomas **Q5** What is the differential diagnosis for a palpable mass?

8	• Palpate for hepatomegaly
	• Start in right iliac fossa (RIF) and work straight up towards the right costal margin and also into epigastrium
	• Palpate for an abdominal aortic aneurysm (AAA): deep palpation above umbilicus (use two hands)
		• Define size of liver
		• Assess liver edge characteristics
		  • Smooth: fatty infiltration, venous congestion
		  • Craggy/irregular: metastases, cysts
		• Tenderness: hepatitis, right heart failure (RHF)
		• Pulsatile: tricuspid regurgitation (TR)
			Q6 What are the causes of hepatomegaly?

9	• Palpate for splenomegaly • Start in RIF and work diagonally up and left to left costal margin	• Note size of spleen • If you cannot feel the splenic edge, palpate with right hand while left hand placed on patient's left lower ribs pulling forward, or ask patient to lie on right side	• You cannot get above a spleen • Note a palpable spleen always indicates splenomegaly **Q7** What are the causes of splenomegaly?

The abdominal exam: point by point in action

	DO	THINK!	EXAM TIPS
10	• Palpate for kidneys • Starting on the right side, place left hand under patient's back and right hand on abdomen. Ask patient to take a breath in and push up with fingers of left hand; kidney can be felt with right hand • Repeat on other side	• Enlarged kidneys: polycystic kidney disease • Mass under LIF/RIF scar: transplanted kidney	• If signs of renal disease/ transplanted kidney present, look for other signs of chronic renal failure (CRF): arteriovenous fistula, neck scars (central lines, parathyroidectomy), abdominal scars (peritoneal dialysis)
11	• Check for ascites (shifting dullness)	• Ascites: CLD, malignancy, hypoalbuminaemic states, heart failure	• If you are unsure whether shifting dullness is present (i.e., a tensely distended abdomen), feel for a fluid thrill **Q8** What are the causes of ascites?

12	• Auscultate	• Bowel sounds
		  • Absent: peritonitis, ileus
		  • High-pitched, tinkling: obstruction
		• Aortic bruits: atheroma, aneurysm
		• Liver bruits (if liver edge felt): hepatocellular carcinoma (HCC), transjugular intrahepatic portosystemic shunt (TIPSS), arteriovenous malformation (AVM)
		• Renal bruit: renal artery stenosis
			• Listen for 2 minutes before concluding that bowel sounds are absent (unlikely in an exam setting)

13	• Examine legs	• Peripheral oedema: CLD, heart failure, hypoalbuminaemic states • Erythema nodosum: IBD • Pyoderma gangrenosum: IBD	
14	• To complete my exam I would check the hernial orifices and perform a digital rectal examination (see later)	• Always finish with a concluding statement to clearly indicate completion of the exam	

Classic OSCE questions

Q1 Peripheral stigmata of chronic liver disease (CLD)

Hands	Palmar erythema Dupuytren's contracture (alcohol-related liver disease)
Nails	Finger clubbing Leuconychia
Eyes	Jaundice
Torso	Spider naevi Loss of body hair Gynaecomastia
Abdomen	Hepatomegaly (not in advanced cirrhosis) Splenomegaly Caput medusae
Legs	Peripheral oedema Hair loss
General	Bruising

Notes

Q2 Causes of jaundice

Pre-hepatic	Gilbert's syndrome (impaired bilirubin excretion) Haemolysis (increased bilirubin production)
Hepatocellular	Hepatitis • Viruses: Hep A–E, Epstein–Barr virus (EBV), cytomegalovirus (CMV) • Alcohol • Autoimmune • Drugs (paracetamol in overdose, isoniazid, rifampacin) • Non-alcoholic steatohepatitis (NASH/NAFLD) • Genetic: haemochromatosis, Wilson's alpha-1 antitrypsin deficiency
Intrahepatic cholestasis	Primary biliary cirrhosis (PBC), Drugs (e.g., co-amoxiclav, flucloxacillin, chlorpromazine)
Posthepatic/cholestatic	Gallstones (usually painful) Malignant biliary obstruction (usually painless)

Notes

Q3 Identify that scar

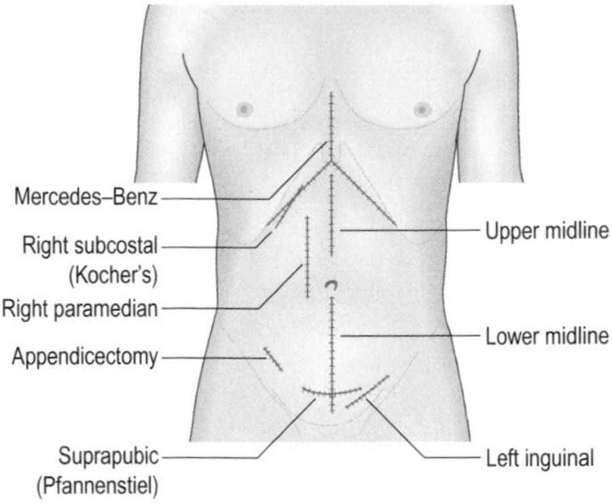

Mercedes–Benz
Right subcostal (Kocher's)
Right paramedian
Appendicectomy
Suprapubic (Pfannenstiel)
Upper midline
Lower midline
Left inguinal

Fig. 3.1 Some abdominal incisions. The midline and oblique incisions avoid damage to innervation of the abdominal musculature and later development of incisional hernias. These incisions have been widely superseded by laparoscopic surgery, however.

Q4 Identify surgical stoma

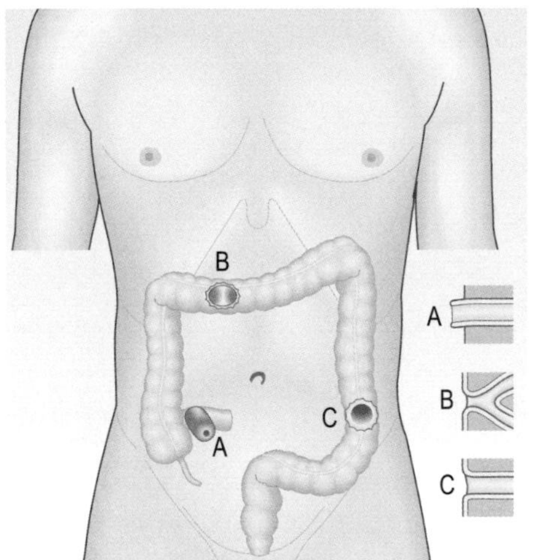

Fig. 3.2 Surgical stomas. A An ileostomy is usually in the right iliac fossa and is formed as a spout. **B** A loop colostomy is created to defunction the distal bowel temporarily. It is usually in the transverse colon and has afferent and efferent limbs. **C** A colostomy may be terminal: that is, resected distal bowel. It is usually flush and in the left iliac fossa.

Notes

Q5 Differential diagnosis of an abdominal mass

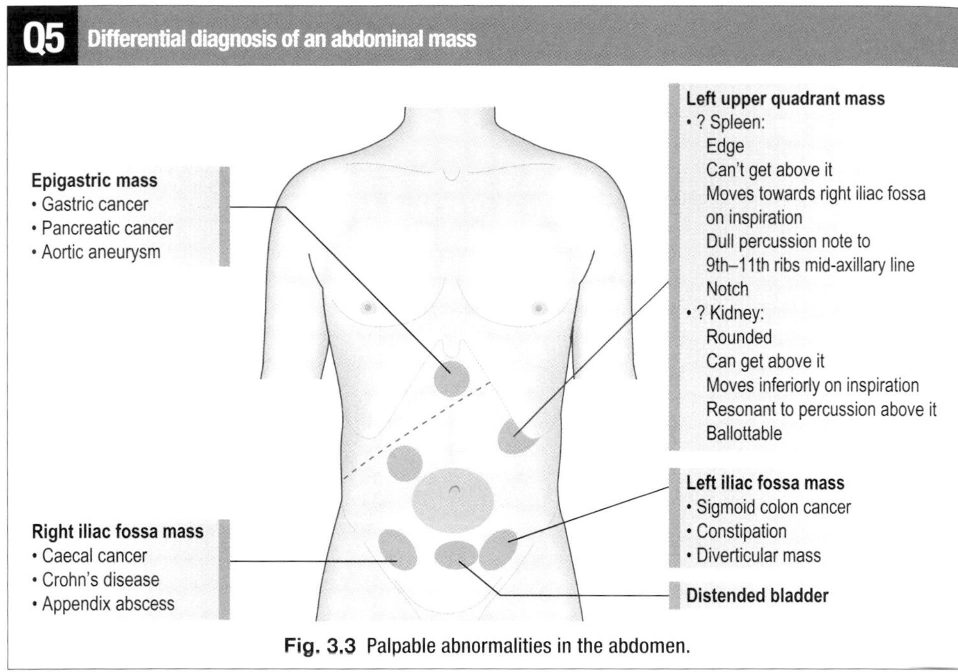

Fig. 3.3 Palpable abnormalities in the abdomen.

Q6 Causes of hepatomegaly

Alcohol	Alcoholic liver disease
Autoimmune	Autoimmune hepatitis
Biliary	Primary biliary cirrhosis
Infections	Viral hepatitis EBV* Malaria*
Infiltrative	Sarcoid* Amyloid* Glycogen storage diseases Hepatic steatosis Haemochromatosis
Haematological	Leukaemia* Lymphoma* Myeloproliferative disorders* e.g., myelofibrosis, polycythaemia rubra vera (PRV) Haemolytic anaemia

Notes

Q6 Causes of hepatomegaly

Malignancy	Hepatocellular carcinoma Metastatic disease
Congestion	RHF Budd–Chiari syndrome TR

*Causes of hepatosplenomegaly
Note liver is shrunken in advanced cirrhosis

Q7 Causes of splenomegaly

Infections	EBV Malaria* Bacterial endocarditis Tuberculosis (TB) Leishmaniasis
Infiltrative	Amyloidosis Sarcoidosis Glycogen storage disease
Haematological	Lymphoma and lymphatic leukaemias e.g., chronic myeloid leukaemia (CML)* Myeloproliferative disease e.g., myelofibrosis* and PRV Haemolytic anaemia
Portal hypertension	
Rheumatological conditions	Rheumatoid arthritis (Felty's syndrome) SLE

*Massive splenomegaly.

Notes

Q8 Causes of ascites

Transudate (protein < 30g/L)	CLD with portal hypertension Budd–Chiari syndrome Hypoalbuminaemia, e.g., nephrotic syndrome, protein-losing enteropathy RHF Constrictive pericarditis (check JVP)
Exudate (protein > 30g/L)	Infection, e.g., spontaneous bacterial peritonitis (SBP), TB (low glucose in ascitic fluid) Malignancy (with peritoneal spread) Pancreatitis (very high amylase in ascitic fluid)

Notes

The digital rectal exam and hernial orifice exam: common OSCE openers

You may be asked to perform a digital rectal examination using a mannikin in an OSCE. Knowing how to do this sensitively but competently and professionally is an important prerequisite of being a doctor.

Common OSCE openers for a hernial orifice exam may include:

1. This patient has noticed a lump in their groin, please examine them
2. This patient is complaining of a fullness in their groin, please examine them

Both examinations follow a simple format as below.

The digital rectal exam and hernial orifice exam: point by point

1 Introduction

2 Inspection

3 Palpation

4 Conclusion

The digital rectal exam: point by point in action

	DO	THINK!	EXAM TIPS
1	• Introduce yourself and a chaperone • Confirm name/DOB • Wash hands and apply gloves • Explain purpose and process of exam • Position patient in left lateral position	• Patient will be anxious and so offer reassurance	• Be professional • Use your full name
2	• Inspect skin and peri-anal region	• Note presence of skin lesions, skin tags, external haemorrhoids, fissures and fistulae	• Fissures/fistulae may indicate IBD
3	• Lubricate index finger with gel • Place pulp of forefinger on anal margin and apply steady pressure on the sphincter to push finger into rectum • Ask patient to squeeze your finger • Palpate systematically around rectum, noting any abnormalities/masses • Identify uterine cervix in women and prostate in men • Assess size, shape, consistency of prostate • Withdraw your finger and examine stool for colour and presence of blood or mucus	• Haemorrhoids ('piles') are congested venous plexuses around the anal canal • Cancer may be palpable as a mucosal irregularity • Lateralised tenderness suggests pelvic peritonitis (unlikely in an exam setting) • Benign prostatic hyperplasia produces palpable symmetrical enlargement. A hard, irregular, asymmetrical prostate with no palpable median groove suggests cancer • Tenderness may indicate prostatitis	• If anal spasm occurs (particularly in anxious patients) ask patient to breath and relax. If necessary, use a local anaesthetic suppository before trying again. • Faecal masses are often palpable but are movable and can be indented

The digital rectal exam: point by point in action

	DO	THINK!	EXAM TIPS
4	• Thank patient • Wash hands	• Allow to dress in private	• If malignancy suspected go on to perform full systematic examination

The hernial orifice exam: point by point in action

	DO	THINK!	EXAM TIPS
	• Introduce yourself • Confirm name/DOB • Wash hands and apply gloves • Examine the groin with the patient standing up	• Hernias are common and occur at openings of the abdominal wall such as the inguinal, femoral and obturator canals, the umbilicus and oesophageal hiatus • The inguinal canal extends from pubic tubercle to anterior superior iliac spine • The femoral canal lies below the inguinal ligament and lateral to the pubic tubercle (Fig. 3.4)	• External hernias are an abnormal protrusion from the abdominal cavity, more obvious when intra-abdominal pressure rises (standing, coughing, sneezing) • Internal hernias occur through defects of the mesentery or into retroperitoneal space and are not visible

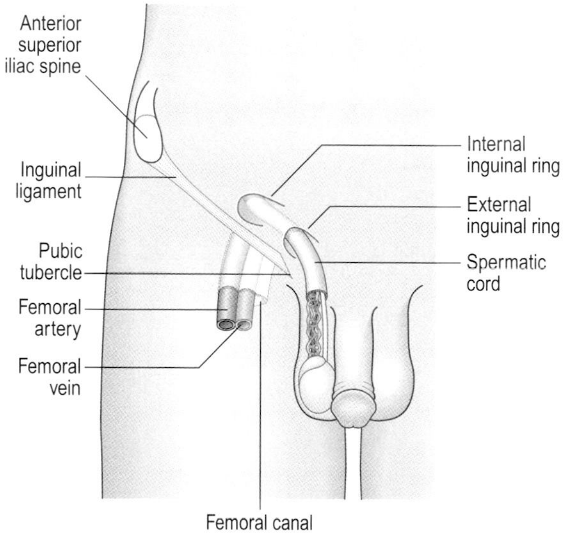

Fig. 3.4 Anatomy of the inguinal canal and femoral sheath.

	DO	THINK!	EXAM TIPS
	• Inspect inguinal and femoral canals and the scrotum for any swellings or lumps • Check for cough impulse		• See page 101 for examination of scrotum

The hernial orifice exam: point by point in action

	DO	THINK!	EXAM TIPS
3	• Palpate the external inguinal ring and along the inguinal canal for muscle defects • Check for a cough impulse • Now ask patient to lie down and assess whether hernia reduces spontaneously. If so, press two fingers over internal inguinal ring at mid-inguinal point and assess cough impulse	• Indirect hernia: hernia does not reappear on coughing with fingers applying pressure over mid-inguinal point • Direct hernia: hernia reappears on coughing with fingers applying pressure over mid-inguinal point • Inguinal hernias are palpable above and medial to pubic tubercle • Femoral hernias are palpable below the inguinal ligament and lateral to the pubic tubercle	• Indirect inguinal hernias comprise 85% of all hernias and are more common in young men • Direct inguinal hernia is more common in older men and women • In a reducible hernia, the contents can be returned to the abdominal cavity • An irreducible hernia may lead to obstruction if it contains bowel or strangulation if the blood supply is restricted (medical emergency) **Q9** Describe the anatomical differences between inguinal and femoral hernias
4	• Thank patient • Wash hands	• Allow to dress	

Q9 Inguinal and femoral hernias

Indirect inguinal hernia	Hernia bulges through the internal ring and follows the course of the inguinal canal. May extend beyond external ring and enter the scrotum
Direct inguinal hernia	Hernia forms at site of muscle weakness in the posterior wall of inguinal canal and rarely extends into scrotum
Femoral hernia	Hernia projects through the femoral ring and into the femoral canal.

Notes

4

The neurological system

Common OSCE openers

1. This patient has weakness of their leg/arm; please examine the lower/upper limbs
2. This patient has had difficulty walking; please examine their lower limbs
3. This patient has noticed altered sensation in their leg/arm; please examine them

The neurological exam: point by point

1 Introduction

2 Inspection

3 Tone

4 Power

5 Reflexes

6 Coordination

7 Sensation

8 Other tests as appropriate

The format above can be used for both lower limb and upper limb examinations. Detailed descriptions of these will follow.

The lower limb neurological exam: point by point in action

	DO	THINK!	EXAM TIPS
1	• Wash hands, introduce yourself • Confirm name/DOB • Check patient not in pain	• Ensure patient adequately exposed • Maintain dignity	• Be professional • Use your full name
2	• Inspect from end of the bed • Inspect proximally and distally	• Asymmetry? (e.g. flexion deformities, pes cavus) • Muscle wasting and fasciculation: lower motor neuron (LMN) lesions • Abnormal movements e.g. myoclonic jerks	• In upper motor neuron (UMN) lesions there is weakness but not wasting **Q1** What are the classical signs of UMN and LMN lesions?
3	• Assess tone • Ask patient to relax and 'go floppy' • Check for pain • Roll the leg from side to side • Briskly flip the knee into the flexed position whilst observing the foot • Check for clonus	• Reduced tone in LMN lesions • Increased tone: spasticity (UMN) or rigidity • Clonus best elicited at ankles • Unsustained (<6 beats) may be physiological; sustained indicates UMN lesion	• Heel typically moves up bed when knee is flipped up. Increased tone may cause it to lift off bed due to failure of relaxation **Q2** What is the difference between spasticity and rigidity?

4	• Assess power
	• Hip flexion/extension
	• Knee flexion/extension
	• Ankle dorsiflexion/plantar flexion
	• Great toe extension
	• Ankle eversion/inversion
		• Assess with patient reclining; compare each movement on one side with the other before moving on. Grade power out of 5
		• Weakness patterns:
		  • Pyramidal weakness (e.g. stroke), extensors weaker than flexors in upper limbs and vice versa in lower limbs
		  • Myopathies: proximal weakness
		  • Neuropathies: distal weakness
		  • Mononeuropathies or radiculopathies: focal weakness (e.g. foot drop caused by common peroneal nerve palsy or L5 radiculopathy)
			• UMN lesions produce weakness of large groups of muscles (e.g. limb)
			• LMN lesions produce weakness of specific muscles
			Q3 Describe the Medical Research Council (MRC) grading of power
			Q4 Describe the nerve and muscle supplies of commonly tested movements

5	• Test reflexes • Test knee jerk and ankle jerk • Test plantar reflex • Use reinforcement if a reflex appears to be absent	• Knee jerk – L3/4 • Ankle jerk – S1 • Plantar reflex – S1/2 • Normal is downward • Up (Babinski) in UMN lesion	• Ensure patient relaxed (anxiety may increase the response) • Compare each reflex with the other side before moving on • Check for symmetry

The lower limb neurological exam: point by point in action			
	DO	**THINK!**	**EXAM TIPS**
6	• Assess coordination • Heel-to-shin test	• Abnormal if heel wavers from line of the shin • In midline cerebellar abnormalities (tumours of vermis, alcoholic cerebellar damage), heel-to-shin may be normal. Truncal ataxia may be only finding	• Weakness may produce false-positive so demonstrate normal power first

7	• Assess sensation
	• Light touch (cotton wool)
	  • Demonstrate on sternum then compare each side in all dermatomes.
	  • If peripheral neuropathy suspected, start distally and look for a glove and stocking pattern. If spinal cord pathology suspected, determine sensory level
	• Superficial pain (neurotip)
	  • Demonstrate on sternum then compare each side in all dermatomes
	• Vibration
	  • Strike tuning fork on own palm. Place on sternum first and repeat on big toe
	  • If absent move proximally to medial malleolus, patella, anterior iliac spine, lower chest wall and clavicle
	  • Repeat on other side and record level at which patient detects vibration
	• Proprioception
	  • With patient's eyes open demonstrate procedure
	  • Repeat with eyes closed comparing each side. If impaired, proceed proximally to metocarpophalangeal (MCP) joint, wrist, elbow, shoulder and clavicle
	• Temperature
	  • Touch patient with cold metallic tuning fork and ask if feels cold
		• See Figure 4.1 for dermatomal and sensory peripheral map innervation
		• Pain and temperature sensation conducted in small, slow-conducting fibres of peripheral nerves and spinothalamic tract. Most pain/ temperature fibres cross to contralateral side on entry to spinal cord
		• Vibration and proprioception are conveyed in large, myelinated fast-conducting fibres in peripheral nerves and posterior columns. Posterior columns remain ipsilateral from point of entry to the spinal cord to the medulla
			• Always ask patient to close their eyes. If they see you touch them, they may say they feel it. 'Dab' cotton wool, don't stroke/tickle
			• It is useful to ask the patient to map out their area(s) of sensory disturbance if they can
			• Ask patient to say yes when they feel you touch their skin. Ask them if it feels the same on both sides.
			• Ankle oedema may affect perception
			• When testing vibration ensure patient feels buzzing, ask patient to close eyes and report when you stop it with your fingers
			• Ensure you hold the sides of the great toe so as not to influence the results
			• Detailed testing of temperature requires hot/cold temperature-controlled water and is rarely performed
			Q5 What is the differential diagnosis for peripheral neuropathy?
			Q6 What are the signs and symptoms of spinal cord compression?

The lower limb neurological exam: point by point in action

	DO	THINK!	EXAM TIPS
	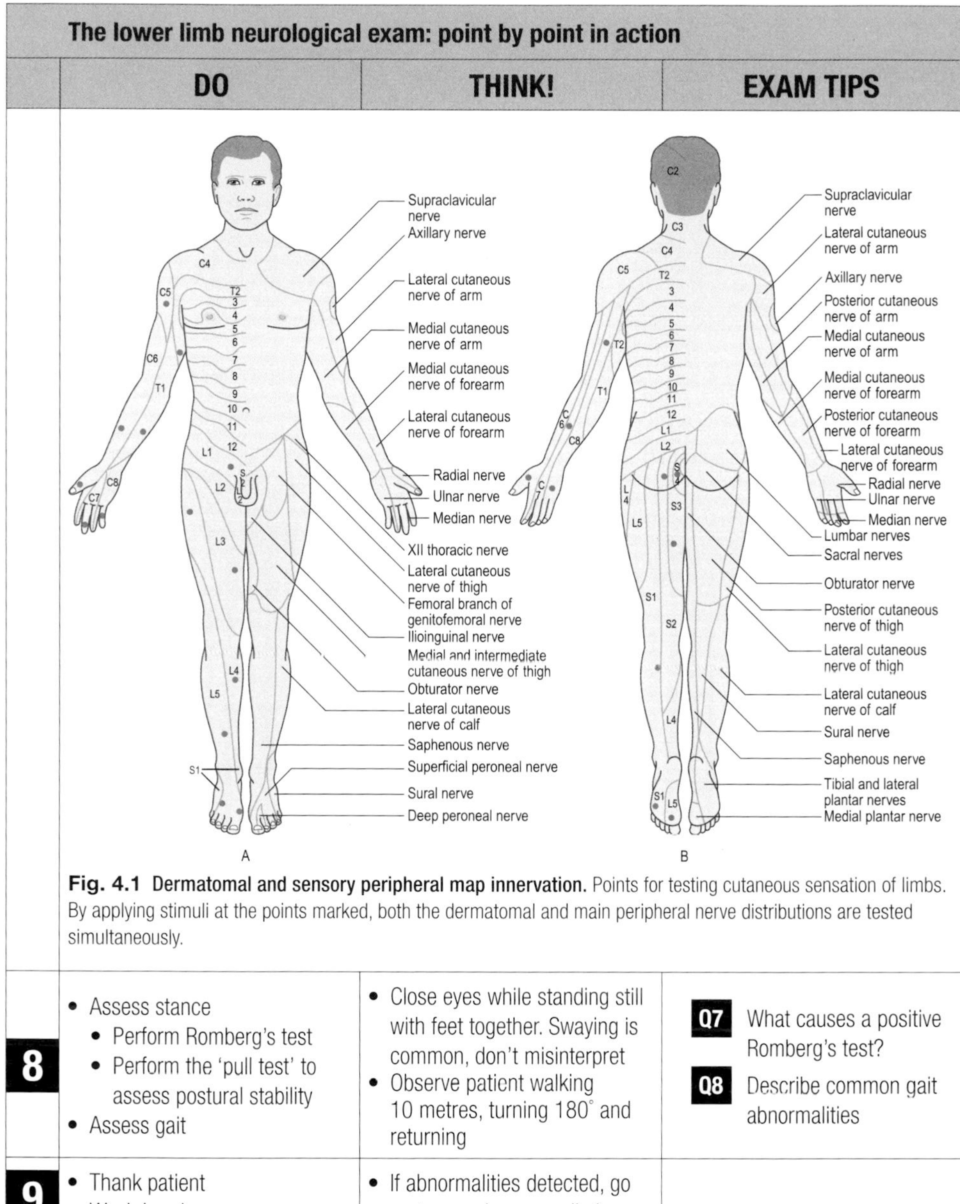 **Fig. 4.1 Dermatomal and sensory peripheral map innervation.** Points for testing cutaneous sensation of limbs. By applying stimuli at the points marked, both the dermatomal and main peripheral nerve distributions are tested simultaneously.		

8	• Assess stance
	  • Perform Romberg's test
	  • Perform the 'pull test' to assess postural stability
	• Assess gait
		• Close eyes while standing still with feet together. Swaying is common, don't misinterpret
		• Observe patient walking 10 metres, turning 180° and returning
			Q7 What causes a positive Romberg's test?
			Q8 Describe common gait abnormalities

9	• Thank patient • Wash hands	• If abnormalities detected, go on to examine upper limbs	

Classic OSCE questions

Q1 Classical signs of UMN and LMN lesions

	UMN lesion	LMN lesion
Inspection	Usually normal (disuse wasting in longstanding lesions)	Muscle wasting Fasciculations
Tone	Increased tone Clonus	Normal/ decreased No clonus
Weakness	Preferentially affects extensors in arms, flexors in legs	Usually more focal in distribution of nerve root or peripheral nerve
Reflexes	Increased	Reduced/absent
Plantar response	Extensor (Babinski sign)	Flexor

Q2 Spasticity vs rigidity

Spasticity	Velocity-dependent resistance to passive movement Pronounced with quick movements UMN sign associated with weakness, hyper-reflexia and extensor plantar responses In severe cases may limit range of movement and be associated with contractures
Rigidity	Sustained resistance throughout range of movement Most easily detected when limb moved slowly In parkinsonism, rigidity is described as 'lead-pipe' and, in the presence of tremor, 'cog-wheeling'

Notes

Q3 Medical Research Council (MRC) grading of muscle power

0	No muscle contraction visible
1	Flicker of contraction but no movement
2	Joint movement when effect of gravity eliminated
3	Movement against resistance but weaker than normal
4*	Movement against resistance but weaker than normal
5	Normal power

*May be further classified as 4+ or 4−

Q4 Nerve and muscle supplies of commonly tested movements

Movement	Muscle	Nerve	Root
Hip flexion	Iliopsoas	Iliofemoral nerve	L1/2
Hip extension	Gluteus maximus	Sciatic	L5/S1
Knee flexion	Hamstrings	Sciatic	S1
Knee extension	Quadriceps	Femoral	L3/4
Ankle dorsiflexion	Tibialis anterior	Deep peroneal	L4/5
Ankle plantar flexion	Gastrocnemius and soleus	Tibial	S1/2
Great toe extension	Extensor hallucis longus	Deep peroneal	L5
Ankle eversion	Peronei	Superficial peroneal	L5/S1
Ankle inversion	Tibialis posterior	Tibial	L4/5

Notes

Q5 Causes of a peripheral neuropathy

Drugs	Isoniazid Nitrofurantoin Amiodarone Phenytoin Chemotherapy (e.g. vincristine, cisplatin)
Metabolic	Diabetes mellitus Chronic kidney disease Hypothyroidism
Nutritional	Vitamin B_{12} deficiency Vitamin B_6 deficiency Vitamin B_1 deficiency Vitamin E deficiency
Toxins	Alcohol Heavy metals (lead, mercury, arsenic)
Infections	Lyme disease EBV Hepatitis C HIV
Malignancy	Leukaemia Lymphoma Paraneoplastic
Connective tissue disease	SLE
Vasculitis	Polyarteritis nodosa

Notes

Q6 Spinal cord compression

Causes	Disc/vertebral lesions (e.g. degeneration, prolapse, trauma, bony metastases) Spinal cord tumours: primary or secondaries (metastases) Inflammatory (e.g. epidural abscess, TB) Extramedullary (e.g. meningioma, neurofibroma) Intramedullary (e.g. ependymoma, glioma)
Symptoms	Back pain Spastic paraparesis below level of lesion Sensory loss below level of lesion (look for sensory level) Zone of hyperaesthesia in dermatomes immediately above level Urinary/faecal incontinence, urinary retention Lhermitte's phenomenon

Notes

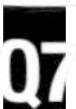

Q7 Romberg's sign

Positive Romberg's sign indicates proprioceptive sensory loss (sensory ataxia).
Cerebellar ataxia is not associated with a positive Romberg's sign. These patients will have difficulty balancing even with eyes open.

Causes of sensory ataxia	
Dorsal column loss	Vitamin B_{12} deficiency (subacute combined degeneration of the spinal cord [SCDC]) Tabes dorsalis (neurosyphilis) Multiple sclerosis
Sensory peripheral neuropathy	Chronic inflammatory demyelinating polyradiculoneuropathy (CIDP)

Q8 Common gait abnormalities

Gait	Description	Causes
Parkinsonian	Stooped posture Slow, shuffling (reduced stride) Loss of arm swing Postural instability Freezing	Parkinson's disease and Parkinsonian syndromes
Gait apraxia	Small, shuffling steps Difficulty in starting Better 'cycling' on bed than walking	Cerebrovascular disease Hydrocephalus
Spastic	Stiff or scissors gait	Spinal cord lesions
Myopathic	Proximal weakness causes a waddling gait Bilateral Trendelenburg sign (see page 63)	Muscular dystrophies and acquired myopathies
Foot drop	Foot slapping	Neuropathies Common peroneal nerve palsy L5 radiculopathy
Central ataxia	Wide-based gait 'Drunk'	Cerebellar disease
Sensory ataxia	Wide-based gait Positive Romberg's sign	Neuropathies Spinal cord lesions
Functional	Variable Often bizarre Inconsistent Dragging immobile leg behind	Functional disorders

The upper limb neurological exam: point by point in action			
	DO	**THINK!**	**EXAM TIPS**
1	• Wash hands, introduce yourself • Confirm name/DOB • Check patient not in pain	• Ensure patient adequately exposed • Maintain dignity	• Be professional • Use your full name
2	• Inspect from end of the bed • Inspect proximally and distally	• Asymmetry? • Muscle wasting or fasciculation (LMN)? • Abnormal movements, e.g. tremor or jerks?	• Tremor is an involuntary, oscillatory movement around a joint caused by alternating contraction/relaxation of muscles **Q1** What are the different kinds of tremor?
3	• Assess tone • Ask patient to relax and 'go floppy' • Check for pain • Hold patient's hand as if shaking hand and support elbow • Use supination/pronation and flexion/extension movements to assess tone at wrist/elbow • Asscss synkinesis by asking patient to move contralateral arm in circular movements in air • Ask patient to make a fist then relax and open hand – watch speed	• Synkinesis used to exaggerate hypertonia particularly in extrapyramidal disease • Myotonia: inability of muscles to relax normally (e.g. myotonic dystrophy, see Chapter 12)	• Transient increase in tone with synkinesis may be normal
4	• Assess power • Shoulder abduction • Elbow flexion/extension • Wrist extension • Finger extension/flexion • Finger abduction • Thumb abduction	• Compare each movement on one side with the other before moving on. Grade power out of 5 • UMN lesions preferentially affect extensors in arms	**Q2** Describe the nerve and muscle supplies of commonly tested movements **Q3** What is the differential diagnosis for a hemiplegia?
5	• Assess reflexes • Test the biceps, triceps and supinator reflexes • Use reinforcement if necessary	• Biceps jerk – C5/6 • Triceps jerk – C7 • Supinator jerk – C5/6	• Strike finger palpating biceps and supinator tendons otherwise painful. Strike triceps tendon itself • To reinforce upper limb reflexes, ask patient to make fist with contralateral hand

The upper limb neurological exam: point by point in action

	DO	THINK!	EXAM TIPS
6	• Assess coordination • Finger-to-nose test • Rapid alternating movements to demonstrate dysdiadochokinesis • 'Piano playing'	• Past pointing (dysmetria)/ intention tremor: cerebellar ataxia • Dysdiadochokinesis: cerebellar ataxia • Piano playing is difficult with UMN lesions, Parkinson's disease	• Hold finger at extreme of patient's reach • Ask patient to repeat the movement as quickly as possible • Change position of target finger

7	• Assess sensation
	• Light touch
	  • Demonstrate on sternum then compare each side in all dermatomes
	  • If peripheral neuropathy suspected, start distally and look for a glove and stocking pattern. If spinal cord pathology suspected, determine sensory level
	• Superficial pain (neurotip)
	  • Repeat above for pain
	• Vibration
	  • Strike tuning fork on own palm
	  • Place on sternum first and repeat on distal interphalangeal (DIP) joint of forefinger
	  • If absent, move proximally to MCP joints, wrist, elbow, shoulder and clavicle
	  • Repeat on other side
	• Proprioception
	  • With patient's eyes open, demonstrate procedure
	  • Repeat with eyes closed comparing each side
	• Temperature
	  • Touch patient with cold metallic tuning fork and ask if it feels cold
		• See Fig. 4.1 for dermatomal and sensory peripheral map innervation
		• When testing vibration, ensure the patient feels buzzing, ask patient to close eyes and report when you stop it with your fingers
			• Always ask patient to close eyes. If they see you touch them, they may say they feel it. 'Dab' cotton wool, don't stroke/tickle
			• Ask patient to say yes when they feel you touch their skin. Ask them if it feels the same on both sides.
			• No need to move proximally if distal sensation intact
			• Detailed testing of temperature requires hot/cold temperature-controlled water and is rarely performed

Classic OSCE questions

Q1 Tremor

Physiological	Fine, fast postural tremor (low amplitude, high frequency) Similar tremor in hyperthyroidism, excess alcohol, caffeine
Essential	Symmetrical in upper limbs, may also involve head and voice Tremor present on posture and with movement May be improved by alcohol Autosomal dominant inheritance
Parkinson's	Slow, coarse, 'pill rolling' tremor Worse at rest, reduced by movement Usually asymmetrical, more common in upper limbs Does not affect the head
Intention	Absent at rest, maximal on movement and on approaching target
Flapping	Hepatic encephalopathy CO_2 retention flap

Notes

Q2 Nerve and muscle supplies of commonly tested movements

Movement	Muscle	Nerve	Root
Shoulder abduction	Deltoid	Axillary	C5
Elbow flexion	Biceps Brachioradialis	Musculocutaneous Radial	C5/C6 C6
Elbow extension	Triceps	Radial	C7
Wrist extension	Extensor carpi radialis longus	Posterior interosseous	C6
Finger extension	Extensor digitorum communis	Posterior interosseous	C7
Finger flexion	Flexor pollicis longus (thumb) Flexor digitorum profundus (index & middle fingers) Flexor digitorum profundus (ring & little fingers)	Anterior interosseous Anterior interosseous Ulnar	C8 C8 C8
Finger abduction	First dorsal interosseous	Ulnar	T1
Thumb abduction	Abductor pollicis brevis	Median	T1

Q3 Causes of hemiplegia (UMN lesion)

Vascular	Stroke: thrombosis, embolism or haemorrhage
Malignancy	Tumours may produce signs depending on site False localising signs occur in the presence of raised intracranial pressure (ICP) (e.g. VI nerve palsy) Papilloedema usually present if raised ICP
Demyelinating disease	Multiple sclerosis
Infection	Cerebral abscesses and mycotic aneurysms may cause hemiplegia

Notes

The cranial nerve exam: common OSCE openers

1. Please examine this patient's cranial nerves (CN)
2. This patient has noticed a change in their vision; please examine their CN
3. This patient has noticed a change in the appearance of their face; please examine them

The cranial nerve exam: point by point

CN I	Olfactory	Sense of smell
CN II	Optic	Visual acuity Visual fields Pupillary reflexes (also CN III) Pupil size and shape Fundoscopy
CN III	Oculomotor	Eye position and movements
CN IV	Trochlear	
CN VI	Abducens	
CN V	Trigeminal	Facial sensation Muscles of mastication Jaw jerk Corneal reflex
CN VII	Facial	Facial expression Taste (anterior 2/3 tongue)
CN VIII	Vestibulo-cochlear	Hearing Rinne/Weber test
CN IX	Glosso-pharyngeal	Pharyngeal sensation (not routinely tested)
CN X	Vagus	Palate movements
CN XI	Spinal accessory	Trapezius and sternomastoid muscles
CN XII	Hypoglossal	Tongue appearance and movement

The cranial nerve exam: point by point in action

	DO	THINK!	EXAM TIPS
General intro	• Wash hands, introduce yourself • Confirm name/DOB	• Position patient sitting opposite at same height	• Be professional • Use your full name
CN I	• Ask the patient if they have noticed a change in their sense of smell	• Hyposmia/anosmia may occur in upper respiratory tract infection, sinus disease, head injury (damage to olfactory filaments), local compression (olfactory groove meningioma), invasion of basal skull tumours	• Disturbances in smell may occur early in Parkinson's and Alzheimer's disease. Altered taste may also be noted

CN II	• Visual acuity
	  • Ideally use Snellen chart
	  • Otherwise ask patient to read something covering one eye at a time
	• Pupils and pupil reflexes
	  • Inspect for anisocoria, ptosis and squint
	  • Check direct and consensual responses
	  • Check for relative afferent pupillary defect (RAPD) by moving light rapidly between eyes
	• Visual fields
	  • Move hat pin towards the centre from four corners of vision
	• Fundoscopy
	  • Often missed out in cranial nerve (CN) exam but say that you would do
		• Ask patients to wear glasses if they usually wear them. Near/reading glasses should only be worn when testing vision
		• RAPD occurs when disease of the retina or optic nerve reduces the response of the eye to light. In normal patients, swinging a light between the eyes causes constriction of both pupils. In RAPD, light in the affected eye causes weaker constriction (apparent dilation)
			• If anisocoria is greater in brighter lighting, then it is the larger pupil that is abnormal. If anisocoria is greater in dim lighting, the smaller pupil is the abnormal one.
			• An equal degree of anisocoria in all levels of lighting indicates physiological anisocoria (20% of population)
			Q1 Describe the causes of anisocoria
			Q2 Describe common visual field defects
			Q3 What is Adie's pupil and Argyll Robertson pupil?

The cranial nerve exam: point by point in action			
	DO	**THINK!**	**EXAM TIPS**

CN III
CN IV
CN VI
	• Observe position of eyes
	  • Look for symmetrical reflection of light on cornea
	• Eye movements
	  • Move finger in 'H' pattern
	  • Ask if patient sees double
	  • Look for nystagmus
	• Accommodation reflex
	  • Observe pupils constricting as you move finger towards nose
		• The eyes are normally parallel in all positions except for convergence
		• Any misalignment where visual axes fail to meet at fixation point is referred to as a squint (strabismus)
		• Lesions of CN III, IV and VI cause abnormal positioning of the eye with diplopia due to weak extraocular muscles. Look for abnormal head posture such as head tilts (CN IV palsy) or head turns (CN VI palsy) – these signs may be subtle
		• Nystagmus is continuous, uncontrolled movement of eyes. It must be sustained for more than a few beats to be significant. Direction of fast phase designates the direction of nystagmus
			Q4 Describe the muscles and innervating nerves involved in the control of eye movements
			Q5 Describe the causes and clinical features of CN III, IV and VI palsies

CN V	• Sensory
	  • Compare light touch sensation on both sides of areas V_1 (ophthalmic), V_2 (maxillary) and V_3 (mandibular)
	• Motor
	  • Clench teeth and feel masseters
	  • Open jaw against force
	  • Note any deviation of jaw
	• Reflexes
	  • Corneal reflex (rarely done)
	  • Jaw jerk
		• V_1: sensation to skin of upper nose, upper eyelid, forehead, scalp, as well as eye and sphenoid/ethmoid sinuses
		• V_2: sensation to upper mouth, pharynx, gums, teeth, palate
		• V_3: floor of mouth, sensation (not taste) anterior ⅔ tongue, lower jaw
		• Motor fibres innervate muscles of mastication (temporalis, masseter, pterygoids)
			• CN V lesions cause unilateral sensory loss on the face and tongue
			• If motor fibres are damaged, jaw deviates to side of lesion when open
			Q6 What is trigeminal neuralgia?

The cranial nerve exam: point by point in action

	DO	THINK!	EXAM TIPS

CN VII	• Inspect face for asymmetry
	• Note differences in blinking and eye closure
	• Ask patient to copy facial moves:
	  • Raise eyebrows, observe forehead (frontalis muscle)
	  • Screw eyes shut, resist opening (orbicularis oculi)
	  • Bear teeth (orbicularis oris)
	  • Blow out cheeks with mouth closed (buccinators and orbicularis oris)
		• Motor supply to muscles of facial expression Parasympathetic fibres to lacrimal, submandibular and sublingual salivary glands. Taste from anterior ⅔ tongue
		• Unilateral LMN CN VII lesion: weakness of both upper and lower facial muscles
		• Unilateral UMN CN VII lesion: weakness of lower facial muscles with relative sparing of upper face. Due to bilateral cortical innervation of upper facial muscles. Eye closure usually preserved
			• Exam usually just motor function, taste rarely tested
			• Minor facial asymmetry is common and benign
			• Causes of LMN CN VII lesion: Bell's palsy, cerebellopontine angle tumour (acoustic neuroma), trauma, parotid tumour, herpes zoster (Ramsay Hunt), sarcoidosis (commonly bilateral), Lyme disease, HIV
			• Causes of UMN CN VII lesion: stroke, tumour
			Q7 What is Bell's palsy?
			Q8 What is Ramsay Hunt syndrome?

CN VIII	• Assess hearing by whispering numbers in one ear while rubbing tragus of other ear then swap sides and repeat
	• Additional special tests:
	  • Weber's test
	  • Rinne's test
		• Clinical features of a cochlear nerve lesion: deafness and tinnitus
		• Vestibular nerve lesions: vertigo and nystagmus
		• This is a crude assessment of hearing
			• Causes of vertigo
			  • Peripheral: labyrinth pathology (e.g. Meniere's disease, vestibular neuronitis, Benign positional vertigo (BPV)), cerebellopontine angle lesions, drugs (e.g. aminoglycosides)
			  • Central: brainstem or cerebellar pathology, e.g. tumours, infarction, MS
			Q9 Describe Weber's and Rinne's tests

The cranial nerve exam: point by point in action			
	DO	**THINK!**	**EXAM TIPS**
CN IX **CN X**	• Assess speech for dysarthria/dysphonia • Ask patient to say 'ah' and look at palate and uvula • Testing pharyngeal sensation unpleasant – instead perform swallow test of water	• Both CNs contain sensory, motor and autonomic components • Main clinical functions include swallowing, phonation, sensation from pharynx/larynx • When saying 'ah' both sides of palate elevate symmetrically and uvula remains in the midline. • Unilateral CN X lesion causes reduced elevation with deviation of uvula away from side of lesion • Bilateral CN X lesions cause dysphagia and dysarthria	• Unilateral CN IX and CN X lesions most commonly caused by stroke, skull base fractures, tumours
CN XI	• Inspect sternomastoid muscles for wasting/hypertrophy • Palpate to assess bulk • Ask patient to shrug shoulders and apply downward pressure (trapezius) • Test power in left side by asking patient to turn to right while you try to resist (sternomastoids). Reverse procedure to check right side	• Isolated CN XI lesions are rare • Possible causes include surgery in posterior triangle of neck, penetrating injuries or tumours	• Wasting of upper fibres of trapezius may be associated with displacement (winging) of scapula away from spine • Wasting/weakness of sternomastoids characteristic of myotonic dystrophy
CN XII	• Inspect tongue for wasting, fasciculation or involuntary movement • Assess whether the tongue deviates on protrusion • Move tongue from side to side • Press tongue against inside of cheek	• Unilateral LMN CN XII lesions cause wasting on affected side and deviation of tongue towards side on protrusion • Bilateral LMN CN XII lesion causes global wasting with a thin, shrunken tongue • Unilateral UMN CN XII lesions are uncommon • Bilateral CN XII lesions lead to spastic tongue and patient can't flick tongue from side to side	**Q10** Describe the features of bulbar and pseudobulbar palsy

Classic OSCE questions

Q1 Causes of anisocoria

Dilated pupil	Cranial nerve III palsy Pharmacological (e.g. tropicamide or atropine) Physiological Post-surgical Adie's tonic pupil
Constricted pupil	Horner's syndrome Pharmacological (e.g. pilocarpine) Physiological Late-stage Adie's tonic pupil

Q2 Visual field defects

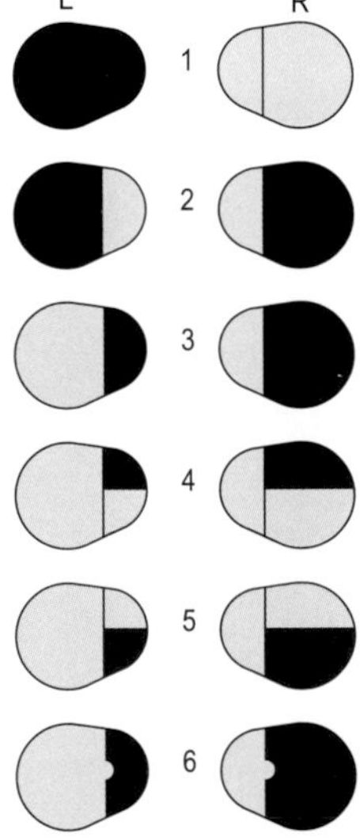

Fig. 4.2 Visual field defects. 1, Total loss of vision in one eye because of a lesion of the optic nerve. 2, Bitemporal hemianopia due to compression of the optic chiasm. 3, Right homonymous hemianopia from a lesion of the optic tract. 4, Upper right quadrantanopia from a lesion of the lower fibres of the optic radiation in the temporal lobe. 5, Lower quadrantanopia from a lesion of the upper fibres of the optic radiation in the anterior part of the parietal lobe. 6, Right homonymous hemianopia with sparing of the macula due to a lesion of the optic radiation in the occipital lobe.

Notes

Q3 Adie's pupil and argyll robertson pupil

Adie's pupil	Benign phenomenon typically affecting young women Mid-dilated pupils responding poorly to light and accommodation With time the affected pupil becomes constricted Holmes–Adie syndrome describes Adie's pupil associated with diminished Achilles tendon reflexes
Argyll Robertson pupil	Pupil is small and irregular Reacts to accommodation but not light Associated with neurosyphilis Other potential causes include diabetes mellitus, optic nerve disease, midbrain lesions

Notes

Q4 Extraocular muscles

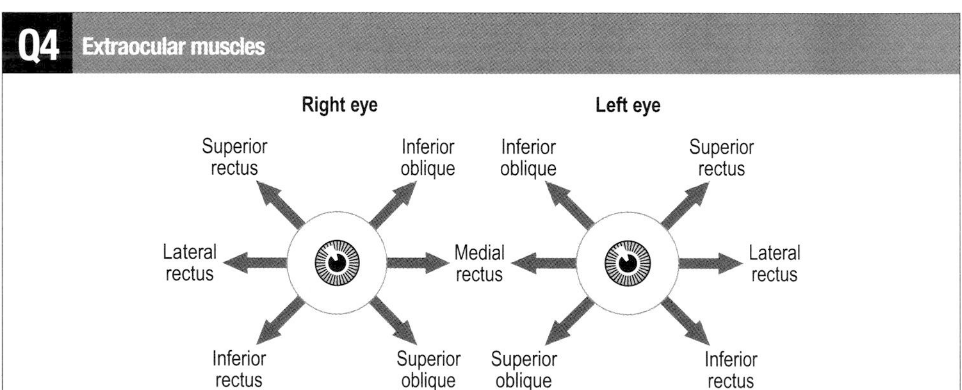

Fig. 4.3 Control of eye movements. Figure illustrates the direction of displacement of the pupil by normal contraction of a particular muscle. It can be used to work out which eye muscle is paretic. For example, a patient whose diplopia is maximum on looking down and to the right has either a weak right inferior rectus or a weak left superior oblique.

Q5 Lesions of CN III, IV, VI

	Clinical features	Causes
CN III	Unilateral complete ptosis Eye facing down and out Fixed and dilated pupil (sparing of pupil means parasympathetic fibres remain undamaged)	Aneurysm of posterior communicating artery (usually painful) Infarction of CN III due to diabetes (pupil usually spared) Infarction of CN III due to atheroma Midbrain infarction/tumour Cavernous sinus pathology, e.g. tumours, internal carotid artery aneurysms Orbital pathology
CN IV	Vertical misalignment of eyes Head tilted away from side of lesion to improve vertical misalignment	Isolated CN IV lesions are rare Head trauma most common acquired cause Cavernous sinus/orbital pathology
CN VI	Affected eye cannot abduct beyond midline Convergent squint with diplopia maximal on looking to side of lesion	Many causes due to long course of nerve Raised ICP Multiple sclerosis Pontine glioma Nasopharyngeal carcinoma Infarction due to diabetes Head trauma Cavernous sinus/orbital pathology

Notes

Q6 Trigeminal neuralgia

Cause	Unknown Almost always unilateral
Clinical features	Severe paroxysms of pain occurring in distribution of CN V Commonly starts in mandibular (V3) and spreads to maxillary (V2) and ophthalmic (V1) Stereotyped, following stimulation of specific trigger zone in face Characteristically doesn't occur at night
Signs	No sign of CN V dysfunction Diagnosis on history alone
Treatment	Avoid triggers Simple analgesia (e.g. paracetamol) Carbamazepine Other agents (e.g. pregabalin) Rarely surgery

Q7 Bell's palsy

Clinical features	LMN CN VII palsy Occasional loss of taste anterior ⅔ tongue
Cause	Considered viral (herpes simplex)
Treatment	Adhesive tape to close eye Steroids (reduce proportion left with deficit) Aciclovir no proven benefit

Notes

Q8 Ramsay Hunt syndrome

Clinical features	LMN CN VII palsy Herpetic vesicles in external auditory meatus Buccal ulceration and ipsilateral loss of taste Occasionally deafness or CN V lesion may occur
Cause	Viral (herpes zoster) infection of geniculate ganglion
Treatment	Aciclovir

Q9 Weber's and Rinne's tests

The purpose of using these tests is to differentiate between conductive and sensorineural hearing loss	
Weber's test	Place vibrating tuning fork in middle of patient's forehead Record which side sound lateralises to if not central Sound should be heard in the middle between both ears In conductive hearing loss, the sound is heard louder in the affected ear In unilateral sensorineural hearing loss it is heard louder in the unaffected ear If symmetrical hearing loss, it will be heard in the middle
Rinne's test	Place vibrating tuning fork on mastoid process Now place vibrating tuning fork in front of ear Ask patient if sound louder in front of ear or behind Normally, sound is louder at external auditory meatus as air conduction is better than bone conduction (Rinne-positive) In conductive hearing loss, bone conduction is better than air conduction (sound louder when tuning fork on mastoid process) (Rinne-negative)
Weber's test is more sensitive and so tuning fork will lateralise to affected ear in conductive hearing loss before Rinne's test becomes abnormal	

Notes

Q10 Bulbar and pseudobulbar palsy

	Bulbar palsy	Pseudobulbar palsy
Motor lesion	LMN lesions of CN IX, X, XI, XII	UMN lesions of CN IX, X, XI, XII
Speech	Dysarthria	Dysarthria and dysphonia
Swallowing	Dysphagia	Dysphagia
Tongue	Wasted and fasciculating	Spastic, slow moving
Jaw jerk	Absent	Brisk
Causes	Motor neuron disease, Guillain–Barré syndrome	Cerebrovascular disease, motor neuron disease, MS

Notes

5

The musculoskeletal system

Common OSCE openers

1. Please perform a GALS screen
2. Please examine this patient's hip/knee/elbow, etc
3. This patient complains of hip/knee/elbow pain when performing tasks; please examine them

The GALS screening exam: point by point

The GALS (gait, arms, legs, spine) is a rapid screen for any musculoskeletal and neurological deficit, whilst also assessing functional ability. It would commonly be used as a broad screening tool before going on to examine particular joints in more detail.

1 Introduction

2 Gait

3 Arms

4 Legs

5 Spine

6 Conclusion

The GALS screening exam: point by point in action

	DO	THINK!	EXAM TIPS
1	• Wash hands, introduce yourself • Confirm name/DOB • Ask initial screening questions: 1. Do you have any pain/ stiffness in your muscles, joints or back? 2. Do you have difficulty dressing yourself? 3. Do you have difficulty walking up and down stairs? 4. Ask patient to undress to their underwear and stand in front of you	• If answers to questions are negative the patient is unlikely to have significant musculoskeletal problems • Maintain patient dignity at all times	• The GALS screen is used to help identify joints that require more detailed examination
2	• Ask patient to walk ahead in a straight line – turn – walk back towards you	• Is the gait symmetrical? • Is there smoothness of movement? • Is the step height normal?	• For common gait abnormalities see page 43
3	• **Look** • Stand in front of patient • Inspect hands, wrists, elbows, shoulders • **Feel** • Squeeze metacarpophalangeal (MCP) joints • Palpate elbows • **Move – ask patient to:** • Clench fists and open hands flat • Squeeze your fingers • Touch each fingertip with thumb • Make a prayer sign and reverse the maneouvre • Put arms straight out in front of body • Bend arms to touch shoulders • Place elbows at side of body bent at 90°, turn palms up and down • Place hands behind head • Place hands behind back	• Look for any swelling, erythema, deformity, nodes, muscle wasting at each joint • Feel for warmth and pain (suggests inflammation)	• Demonstrate each action to the patient rather than explaining what to do • Any asymmetry, pain or reduced movement will require a more detailed examination of that joint (see later)

The GALS screening exam: point by point in action

	DO	THINK!	EXAM TIPS

4	• **Look**
	  • Ask patient to lie on couch
	  • Inspect hips, knees, ankles, feet
	• **Feel**
	  • Palpate knees for warmth, swelling, patellar tap
	  • Squeeze metatarsal heads for pain
	• **Move**
	  • Flex each hip and knee to 90°
	  • Passively rotate each hip internally and externally
		• As above look for swelling, erythema, deformity, asymmetry
		• Look at soles of feet for calluses and ulcers
		• Feel for crepitus in the patellofemoral joint and knee
			• Consider performing Thomas's test for fixed flexion deformity (see later)

5	• **Look**
	  • Examine spine from back, front, side
	• **Feel**
	  • Stand behind patient and hold their pelvis, ask them to turn from side to side without moving feet
	• **Move**
	  • Stand behind and ask patient to slide hand down lateral aspect of thigh
	  • Stand beside patient and ask them to touch toes
	  • Face patient and ask them to touch each ear on shoulder
	  • Ask patient to look down at the floor then up to ceiling
		• Assess straightness of spine, muscle bulk and symmetry
		• Assess for abnormal spinal curvature or limited hip flexion while touching toes
			• Most spinal diseases affect more than one part of the spine and lead to altered posture or function of the spine
			• Low back pain is extremely common and a detailed history and examination is required to elucidate the problem
			Q1 What are the 'red flag' features of acute low back pain?

6	• Thank patient • Allow to dress	• The GALS screen provides a rapid but limited assessment. A more detailed examination is indicated if any abnormalities are detected	

The joint exam: point by point

All joint examinations follow the same basic principles as outlined below with additional specific tests according to the joint involved. The following pages will describe each individual examination following the same principles:

1. Introduction
2. Look
3. Feel
4. Move
5. Special tests
6. Conclusion

The hip exam: point by point in action

DO	THINK!	EXAM TIPS
• Wash hands, introduce yourself • Confirm name/DOB • Check if any pain anywhere	• Ensure patient adequately exposed • Undress to underwear and remove socks and shoes • Should be able to see iliac crests	• Compare affected hip with unaffected hip

• Ask patient to stand
• From front:
  • Inspect stance
  • Compare symmetry of pelvis
  • Check hips, knees, ankles, feet
• From side:
  • Assess lumbar lordosis, stoop
• From behind
  • Assess spine curvature
  • Check positions of shoulders, pelvis
  • Check lengths of leg
  • Assess for gluteal atrophy
	• Look for:
	  • Deformity of joint
	  • Evidence of muscle wasting
	  • Scars
	• Limited hip extension may lead to lumbar lordosis
	• Assess for scoliosis (lateral curvature of spine)
		• Look for mobility aids beside bed
		• Shoulders should lie parallel to ground and symmetrically over pelvis. This may mask a hip deformity or true shortening of the leg

• Palpate hip joint including
  • Greater trochanter
  • Anterior superior iliac crest
	• Warmth and pain suggest inflammation
	• Pain over greater trochanter suggests greater trochanteric pain syndrome (GTPS)
		• GTPS
		  • Inflammation of trochanteric bursa
		  • May be due to injury but often no cause identified
		  • Common in middle-aged women
		  • Treated by relieving aggravating factors, weight loss, exercise, analgesia

• Check range of movement of each hip in turn:
  • Abduction and adduction
  • Internal and external rotation
  • Extension
	• Normal range of movement:
	  • Abduction 45°, adduction 20°
	  • Internal/external rotation 45°
	  • Extension 0–20°
		• Always compare the affected side with the patient's unaffected side as a control

The hip exam: point by point in action

	DO	THINK!	EXAM TIPS

5	• Thomas's test (fixed flexion deformity)
	  • Place hand under patient's back
	  • Passively flex both legs
	  • While keeping non-test hip flexed, ask patient to extend test hip
	• Shortening
	  • Ask patient to lie on couch
	  • Measure from umbilicus to medial malleolus (apparent length)
	  • Measure from anterior superior iliac spine to medial malleolus (true length)
	• Trendelenburg's sign
	  • Stand in front of patient
	  • Palpate both iliac crests and ask patient to stand on each leg for 30 seconds
	  • Assess which iliac crest moves
		• Incomplete extension of test hip indicates fixed flexion deformity
		• By placing your hand beneath patient's back, you can confirm lordotic curve of spine remains eliminated as this may mask hip limitation
		• Shortening may be true or apparent. Apparent shortening is present if the affected limb appears shortened (e.g. adduction or flexion deformity at hip commonly due to OA)
		• Normally, the iliac crest with the foot off the ground should rise
		• Test is positive if unsupported hemipelvis falls below horizontal
			• Do not perform Thomas's test if patient has hip replacement on non-test side; forced flexion may cause dislocation
			Q2 What are the causes of true lower limb shortening?
			• Trendelenburg's sign may be positive when there is gluteal weakness or inhibition from hip pain (osteoarthritis) or structural abnormality of the hip joint

6	• Thank patient • Allow to dress	• Consider further investigations as appropriate (e.g. imaging)	**Q3** What are the indications and complications associated with a total hip replacement?

The knee exam: point by point in action

	DO	THINK!	EXAM TIPS
1	• Wash hands, introduce yourself • Confirm name/DOB • Check if any pain anywhere	• Ensure patient adequately exposed • Undress to underwear and remove socks and shoes	• Complex joint • Depends on muscles and ligaments for stability
2	• Ask patient to lie on couch • Expose legs and examine	• Check for scars, erythema, muscle wasting, swelling • Check for leg length discrepancy • Housemaid's knee: prepatellar bursitis • Baker's cyst: bursa enlargement in popliteal fossa	• If patient lies with one knee flexed the underlying cause may be related to the hip, knee or both

The knee exam: point by point in action

	DO	THINK!	EXAM TIPS
3	• Feel each knee • Palpate medial/lateral joint lines • Patellar tap • Bulge or ripple test	• Check for warmth, compare sides • Patellar tap will elicit tapping sensation when effusion present	• Bulge or ripple test is useful if only a small amount of fluid is present. False negative results may occur if a tense effusion is present

4	• Active flexion/extension
	• Passive flexion/extension
		• Normal range of movement:
		  • Flexion 0–140°
		  • Extension 0° (i.e. flat on couch)
		  • 10° hyperextension normal
			• Restriction to passive extension:
			  • Meniscal tears
			  • Osteoarthritis
			  • Inflammatory arthritis
			• Restriction to passive full flexion (test with patient face down)
			  • Tear of the posterior horn of the menisci

5	• Collateral ligament test:
	  • Fully extend knee
	  • Hold ankle between elbow and side of your body
	  • Apply valgus/varus pressure to knee
	  • Feel joint line and assess degree of joint space opening
	  • Repeat with knee flexed to 30°
	• Cruciate test:
	  • Flex knee to 90°
	  • Use your thigh to immobilise patient's foot
	  • With hands behind upper tibia pull anteriorly
	  • Push backwards on tibia
	• Meniscal tests (McMurray test):
	  • Lie patient supine
	  • Medial meniscus
	    • Passively fully flex knee
	    • Externally rotate foot and abduct upper leg at hip (varus stress at knee)
	    • Extend knee smoothly
	  • Lateral meniscus
	    • Passively fully flex knee
	    • Internally rotate foot and adduct leg at hip (valgus stress at knee)
	    • Extend knee smoothly
	• Patella apprehension test:
	  • Fully extend knee
	  • Push patella laterally and flex knee slowly
		• Opening of joint suggests collateral and cruciate injury
		• Flexing the knee relaxes the cruciate allowing assessment of minor collateral laxity
		• Movement indicates lax anterior cruciate ligament (ACL), movement >1.5 cm suggests rupture
		• Posterior movement suggests posterior cruciate ligament (PCL) laxity
		• In the presence of a medial or lateral meniscus tear, a click is felt on extending the knee, accompanied by discomfort
		• If patient resists flexion, this suggests previous patellar dislocation or instability
			• Abduction or adduction with the knee fully extended should not occur unless lax or ruptured collateral ligament
			• Meniscal injuries in young patients usually occur from twisting injury. In middle-aged patients, degenerative disease is more common with no history of trauma

The knee exam: point by point in action

	DO	THINK!	EXAM TIPS
6	• Thank patient • Allow to dress	• Consider further investigations as appropriate (e.g. imaging)	

The ankle and foot exam: point by point in action

	DO	THINK!	EXAM TIPS
1	• Wash hands, introduce yourself • Confirm name/DOB • Check if any pain anywhere	• Ask patient to remove socks and shoes	• Examine footwear for clues (abnormal pattern of wear, orthotics)

2	• Look at foot and ankle
	• From behind:
	  • Assess alignment of heel
	• From side:
	  • Assess position of midfoot and medial longitudinal arch for pes planus/pes cavus
		• Assess for scars, swelling, deformity, asymmetry, bruising, nail changes, hallux valgus
		• Splay foot:
		  • Widening at level of metatarsal heads suggests metatarsophalangeal (MTP) synovitis
			• Pes planus:
			  • Medial longitudinal arch flattened (flat foot)
			• Pes cavus:
			  • Medial longitudinal arch exaggerated

3	• Feel feet and ankles • Compress midfoot, MTP joints and individual toe joints	• Check for warmth, compare sides • Assess pain	• If feet cool, check peripheral pulses

4	• Active plantar flexion/dorsiflexion
	• Active inversion/eversion of foot
	• Active flexion/extension of toes
	
	• Passive plantar flexion/dorsiflexion
	• Passive inversion/eversion of foot
	• Passive flexion/extension of toes
		• Normal range of movement:
		  • Dorsiflexion 15°
		  • Plantar flexion 45°
		  • Foot inversion 20°
		  • Foot eversion 10°
			• If dorsiflexion restricted, repeat dorsiflexion with knee extended and flexed. If more dorsiflexion possible, suggests gastrocnemius contracture

5	• Achilles tendon
	  • Ask patient to kneel on a chair
	  • Palpate gastrocnemius and Achilles tendon
	• Thomson's (Simmonds') test:
	  • Squeeze calf just distal to level of maximum circumference
		• Achilles tendon rupture may be palpable as a gap in the tendon about 5 cm above calcaneal insertion
		• On squeezing the calf, absence of plantar flexion suggests tendon rupture
			• You are unlikely to be asked to perform this test in an exam as the patient would be in too much pain. However, it is important that you know the process

6	• Thank patient • Allow to dress	• Consider further investigations as appropriate (e.g. imaging)	

The shoulder exam: point by point in action

	DO	THINK!	EXAM TIPS
1	• Wash hands, introduce yourself • Confirm name/DOB • Check if any pain anywhere	• Ask patient to sit or stand but expose shoulder completely	
2	• Examine from front and back • Look in axillae	• Look for swelling, deformity, muscle wasting • Check position of scapula: elevated, depressed, winged	• Shoulder pain is common. May be due to the shoulder itself or referred pain from cervical spine or sub-diaphragmatic via phrenic nerve
3	• Palpate • From sternoclavicular joint along clavicle to acromioclavicular joint • Acromion and coracoid processes, scapula spine and biceps tendon • Supraspinatus tendon	• Check for warmth or erythema • Joint tenderness • Osteophytes	• To palpate supraspinatus tendon, extend the shoulder to bring supraspinatus anterior to acromion process
4	• Active movements • Flexion/extension • Abduction • Internal/external rotation • Deltoid (abduct arm while pushing down humerus)	• Normal range of movement: • Flexion 180°, extension 60° • abduction 180° • internal rotation 90°, external rotation 70–90°	• Abduction: • 0–15° supraspinatus • 15–90° deltoid • >90° trapezius and serratus anterior with scapula rotated
	• Rotator cuff muscles: • Internal rotation (Gerber test) • Place patient's hand behind their back • Ask them to lift hand off back • Abduction of arm • With arm at side test abduction • External rotation • Test with arm in neutral position and at 30° to reduce deltoid contribution	• Rotator cuff muscles • Internal rotation • Subscapularis and pectoralis major • Inability to lift hand off back: tear in subscapularis • Pain: tendonitis • Abduction • Supraspinatus • Loss of power: tear • Pain: tendonitis • External rotation • Infraspinatus and teres minor • Loss of power: tear • Pain: tendonitis	• To test muscles of rotator cuff, effect of other muscles crossing shoulder need to be neutralised so specific movements are required • No movement or fixed internal rotation suggests a frozen shoulder
	• Biceps tendon • Palpate long head of biceps on head of humerus • Ask patient to supinate forearm • Ask patient to flex against resistance	• Pain: biceps tendonitis • Rupture: long head of biceps bulges distally (Popeye sign)	
	• Impingement tests • Passively fully abduct patient's arm • Ask patient to adduct slowly	• Painful arc when pain occurs at 60–120° of abduction (subacromial impingement syndrome)	• Pain on active movement, especially against resistance, suggests impingement

The shoulder exam: point by point in action

	DO	THINK!	EXAM TIPS

5	• Tests for impingement:
	  • Neer test
	    • Patient's elbow fully extended
	    • Scapular rotation prevented with examiner's hand
	    • Abduct arm in internal rotation
	  • Hawkins–Kennedy test
	    • Shoulder flexed at 90°, elbow flexed at 90°
	    • Examiner forcefully rotates arm internally
		• Neer test causes greater tuberosity to impinge against acromion
		• Positive result indicated by pain
		• Positive result in Hawkins-Kennedy test indicated by pain
			Q4 What are common conditions affecting the shoulder?

6	• Thank patient • Allow to dress	• Consider further investigations as appropriate (e.g. imaging)	

The elbow exam: point by point in action

	DO	THINK!	EXAM TIPS
1	• Wash hands, introduce yourself • Confirm name/DOB • Check if any pain anywhere	• Ensure arm exposed from shoulder to hand • Ask patient to stand with arms by their sides and palms forwards	• Elbow pain may be localised or referred from the neck
2	• General inspection • Check alignment of extended elbow	• Check for swelling, nodules (rheumatoid), deformity, rash (psoriasis), tophi	• A valgus angle of 11–13° with the elbow fully extended is normal (carrying angle)

3	• Palpate
	  • Lateral and medial epicondyles
	  • Olecranon bursa
	  • Nodules if present
		• Synovitis suggested by sponginess either side of olecranon when elbow extended	• Rheumatoid nodules may be palpable on the proximal extensor surface of the forearm

4	• Flexion/extension
	• Supination/pronation
		• Normal range of movement:
		  • Flexion/extension 0–145°
		  • Supination 0–90°
		  • Pronation 0–85°
			• A flexion/extension range of less than 30–110° will lead to functional impairment

The elbow exam: point by point in action

	DO	THINK!	EXAM TIPS
5	• Tennis elbow (lateral epicondylitis) • Patient flexes elbow to 90° • Pronate hand & flex hand/wrist fully • Support elbow and ask patient to extend wrist against resistance • Golfer's elbow (medial epicondylitis) • Patient flexes elbow to 90° • Supinate hand fully • Support elbow and ask patient to flex against resistance	• Positive test: pain is produced at the lateral epicondyle, may be referred down extensor aspect of arm • Positive test: pain produced at medial epicondyle, may be referred down flexor aspect of arm	
6	• Thank patient • Allow to dress	• Consider further investigations as appropriate (e.g. imaging)	

The hand exam: point by point in action

	DO	THINK!	EXAM TIPS
1	• Wash hands, introduce yourself • Confirm name/DOB • Check if any pain anywhere	• Seat patient in front of you • Expose arms and shoulders	• Look around the bedside for aids • Look at patient's clothing, e.g. velcro instead of buttons

<table>
<tr><th colspan="4">The hand exam: point by point in action</th></tr>
<tr><th></th><th>DO</th><th>THINK!</th><th>EXAM TIPS</th></tr>
<tr><td>2</td><td>• Examine wrists, hands, fingers, nails</td><td>• Wrists:
  • Scars
  • Swelling/erythema
  • Prominent ulnar styloid: rheumatoid
  • Anterior displacement (partial dislocation): rheumatoid
• Hands
  • Swelling/erythema: synovitis, infection
  • Scars
  • Muscle wasting: inflammatory arthritis, ulnar/median nerve palsy (hypothenar/thenar eminence wasting), T1 nerve root lesions (small muscles of hand)
  • Dupuytren's contracture
  • Palmar erythema
  • Psoriatic plaques
  • Nodules: rheumatoid
  • Skin tight/waxy/cold: scleroderma
• Fingers
  • Deformities, swelling, erythema
  • Subluxation and ulnar deviation of MCP joints: rheumatoid
  • Heberden's (distal interphalangeal [DIP]) and Bouchard (proximal interphalangeal [PIP]) nodes: osteoarthritis
• Nails
  • Pitting, onycholysis: psoriatic arthritis</td><td>• There are many signs to look out for here but practically speaking this is a very concise part of the examination

Q5 Describe different deformities of the fingers</td></tr>
<tr><td>3</td><td>• Palpate above/below interphalangeal joints
• Squeeze MCP joints
• Palpate flexor tendon sheaths in hand</td><td>• Check for tenderness and localise
• Check temperature
• Assess any swelling
• Crepitus may occur with movement of radiocarpal joints in osteoarthritis</td><td>• Hard swellings: bony
• Soft swellings: synovitis</td></tr>
</table>

The hand exam: point by point in action

DO	THINK!	EXAM TIPS

• Active movements
  • Make a fist then extend fingers fully
  • Test flexors/extensors of fingers:
    • Flexor digitorum profundus
    • Flexor digitorum superficialis
    • Extensor digitorum
    • Flexor pollicis longus
    • Extensor pollicis longus
  • Squeeze fingers
  • Prayer sign
  • Reverse prayer sign
  • Check pronation, supination, flexion and extension, ulnar and radial deviation
• Passive movements:
  • Flex/extend each finger/ wrist
	• Finger flexors/extensors (Fig. 5.2)
	  • Flexor digitorum profundus
	    • Ask patient to flex DIP while you hold PIP in extension (Fig. 5.2A)
	  • Flexor digitorum superficialis
	    • Hold patient's other fingers extended and ask patient to flex PIP (Fig. 5.2B)
	  • Extensor digitorum
	    • Ask patient to extend fingers with wrist in neutral position (Fig. 5.2C)
	  • Flexor/extensor pollicis longus
	    • Hold proximal phalanx of patient's thumb and ask them to flex/extend interphalangeal joint (Fig. 5.2D)
	  • Extensor pollicis longus
	    • Ask patient to place palm on flat surface and extend thumb (Fig. 5.2E)
		• In prayer and reverse prayer sign, normal is 90° of extension/flexion

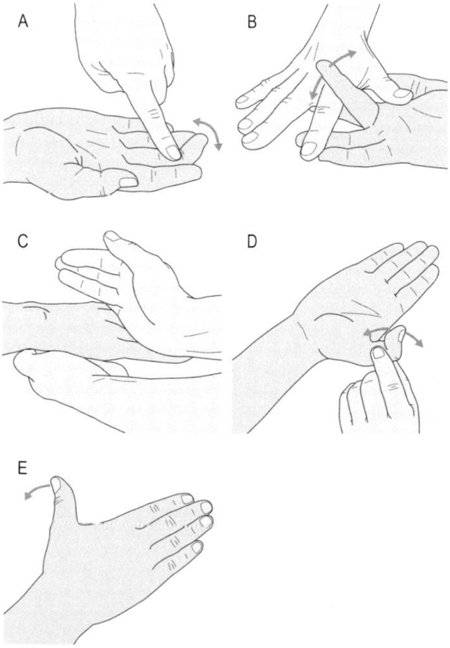

4

A B C D E

Fig. 5.1 Testing the flexors and extensors of the fingers and thumb. A Flexor digitorum profundus. **B** Flexor digitorum superficialis. **C** Extensor digitorum. **D** Flexor pollicis longus. **E** Extensor pollicis longus.

The hand exam: point by point in action

	DO	THINK!	EXAM TIPS

5	• Motor function:
	• Radial nerve
	  • Ask patient to extend wrist and fingers fully; 'paper sign'
	  • Ulnar nerve
	  • Ask patient to make 'scissors sign'
	  • Grip a card placed between their fingers and try to pull it out
	  • Spread fingers against resistance
	• Median nerve
	  • Ask patient to clench fist; 'stone sign'
	  • Also abduct thumb away from palm
	  • Touch thumb and ring finger together and examiner try to pull apart
	  • Ask patient to make the 'OK' sign (anterior interosseous branch)
	
	• Sensory function:
	• Radial nerve
	  • Sensory loss over dorsum of hand and loss of triceps jerk
	• Ulnar nerve
	  • Sensory loss on ulnar side of hand splitting ring finger
	• Median nerve
	  • Sensory loss over hand involving thumb, index, middle finger and lateral aspect ring finger
		• All intrinsic muscles of the hand are innervated by the ulnar nerve except four muscles supplied by median nerve (LOAF):
		  • Lateral 2 lumbricals
		  • Opponens pollicis brevis
		  • Abductor pollicis brevis
		  • Flexor pollicis brevis
		
		• Carpal tunnel syndrome: compression of median nerve as it passes between flexor retinaculum and carpal bones at the wrist
		• Tinel's sign: tapping distal wrist crease with tendon hammer produces tingling in median nerve territory
		• Phalen's test: forced flexion of the wrist up to 60 seconds induces symptoms
			• Use paper – scissors – stone – OK as an aide-memoire
			
			Q6 Describe the common features of carpal tunnel syndrome
			Q7 List the investigations you would perform in a patient with suspected rheumatoid arthritis
			Q8 List the extra-articular manifestations of rheumatoid arthritis

6	• Thank patient • Allow to dress	• Consider further investigations as appropriate (e.g. imaging)	

The spine examination: point by point in action			
	DO	**THINK!**	**EXAM TIPS**
1	• Wash hands, introduce yourself • Confirm name/DOB • Check if any pain anywhere	• Ensure patient's back is fully exposed. Maintain dignity • Ask patient to stand	• Most spinal diseases affect multiple segments causing altered posture or function of the whole spine

2	• Cervical spine
	  • Face the patient and observe posture of head and neck
	• Thoracic/lumbar spine
	  • Observe from behind, side and front
		• Loss of lordosis/increased lordosis/scoliosis
		• Abnormal curvature?
		• Soft tissue abnormalities
			• Soft tissue abnormalities may overlie congenital abnormality, e.g. spina bifida
			• Loss of cervical lordosis occurs with muscle spasm
			• Loss of lumbar lordosis occurs in disorders such as ankylosing spondylitis and disc protrusion

3	• Palpate cervical spine
	  • Midline spinous processes (occiput – T1)
	  • Paraspinal soft tissues
	  • Supraclavicular fossa
	  • Anterior neck including thyroid
	• Palpate thoracic/lumbar spine
	  • Midline spinous processes (T1–T12)
	  • Paraspinal soft tissues
	• Lumbar spine only
	  • Percuss with closed fist noting any tenderness
		• Check alignment of spinous processes
		• Check for prominence of spinal processes
		• Check for pain on palpation of paraspinal soft tissues and muscles
		• Are there nodes or cervical rib in supraclavicular fossa?
			• Be very cautious moving the C-spine in patients with rheumatoid arthritis as atlantoaxial instability can lead to cord damage (unlikely in an OSCE)
			• Prominent spinous process suggests vertebral body collapse
			• Gibbus may also be evident (localised angular flexion of a vertebrae due to anterior wedge deformity)

The spine examination: point by point in action

	DO	THINK!	EXAM TIPS
4	• Cervical spine • Flexion: ask patient to look at the floor • Extension: ask patient to look at the ceiling • Lateral flexion: touch each ear to the ipsilateral shoulder • Lateral rotation: look over each shoulder • Thoracic spine • Rotation: ask patient to sit with arms crossed and twist in both directions and look behind • Lumbar spine: • Forward flexion: ask patient to touch their toes (keep legs straight) • Extension: ask patient to lean back as far as possible • Lateral flexion: reach down to touch outside of each leg (keep legs straight)	• Cervical spine • Normal range of cervical spine movement • Flexion: 0–80° • Extension: 0–50° • Lateral flexion: 0–45° • Lateral rotation: 0–80° • If active movements are reduced, perform passive movements • Thoracic spine • Movement is mainly rotational with limited amount of flexion, extension and lateral rotation • Lumbar spine • Surface markings: L4 (level of pelvic brim) and 'dimples of Venus' (overlie sacroiliac joints) • Normal range of movement: • Flexion: see Schober's test • Extension: 10–20°	• Pain or paraesthesia down the arm on passive neck movement suggests nerve root involvement **Q9** What are the common causes of thoracic spine pain? • Note some of forward flexion at lumbar spine depends on hip flexion and so even with a rigid lumbar spine, forward flexion can still occur if hips are mobile
5	• Schober's test for forward flexion • Mark skin in the midline at L5/level of posterior iliac spines (mark A) • Draw two more marks: one 10 cm above (B) and one 5 cm below this (C) • Ask patient to touch toes and measure from B → C • Distance should increase to >20 cm if forward flexion is normal • Sciatic nerve stretch test • With patient lying supine, lift foot to flex hip passively, keeping knee straight • Raise leg to just less than limit and dorsiflex foot • Femoral nerve stretch test • With patient lying prone, flex knee and extend hip	• Intervertebral disc prolapse causing nerve root pressure occurs most often in the lumbar spine • Problems with femoral nerve roots may cause quadriceps weakness and/or reduced knee jerk reflex • Sciatic nerve (L4–S1) • Limited straight leg raise = positive test • Tension is increased by dorsiflexing the foot (Bragard's test). • Tension is relieved by flexing the knee • Femoral nerve (L2–L4) • Pain in the back or front of thigh = positive test	**Q10** Describe the common causes of low back pain and their associated features **Q11** What are the signs, symptoms and treatment of ankylosing spondylitis?
6	• Thank patient • Allow to dress	• Consider further investigations as appropriate (e.g. imaging)	

Classic OSCE questions

Q1 'Red flag' features for acute low back pain

Features that may indicate serious pathology and require urgent referral

History

- Age < 20 years or > 55 years
- Recent significant trauma (fracture)
- Pain:
  - Thoracic (dissecting aneurysm)
  - Non-mechanical (infection/tumour/pathological fracture)
- Fever (infection)
- Difficulty in micturition
- Faecal incontinence
- Motor weakness
- Sensory changes in the perineum (saddle anaesthesia)
- Sexual dysfunction, e.g. erectile/ejaculatory failure
- Gait change (cauda equina syndrome)
- Bilateral 'sciatica'

Past medical history

- Cancer (metastases)
- Previous glucocorticoid use (osteoporotic collapse)

System review

- Weight loss/malaise without obvious cause, e.g. cancer

Q2 Causes of true lower limb shortening

Hip	• Fractures, e.g. neck of femur • Following total hip arthroplasty • Slipped upper femoral epiphysis • Perthes disease (juvenile osteochondritis) • Unreduced hip dislocation • Septic arthritis • Loss of articular cartilage (arthritis, joint infection) • Congenital coxa vara • Missed congenital dislocation of the hip
Femur and tibia	Growth disturbance secondary to: • Poliomyelitis • Cerebral palsy • Fractures • Osteomyelitis • Septic arthritis • Growth-plate injury • Congenital causes

Notes

Q3 Indications for total hip replacement

Indications	Complications
Osteoarthritis (commonest) Inflammatory arthropathies Displaced intracapsular fracture (in limited circumstances)	Dislocation Infection Peri-operative (anaesthetic, infection, bleeding) Leg length discrepancy

Q4 Common conditions affecting the shoulder

Non-trauma	• Rotator cuff syndromes, e.g. supraspinatus, infraspinatus tendonitis • Impingement syndromes (involving the rotator cuff and subacromial bursa) • Adhesive capsulitis ('frozen shoulder') • Calcific tendonitis • Bicipital tendonitis • Inflammatory arthritis • Polymyalgia rheumatica
Trauma	• Rotator cuff tear • Glenohumeral dislocation • Acromioclavicular dislocation • Fracture of the clavicle • Fracture of the head or neck of the humerus

Notes

Q5 Deformities of the fingers

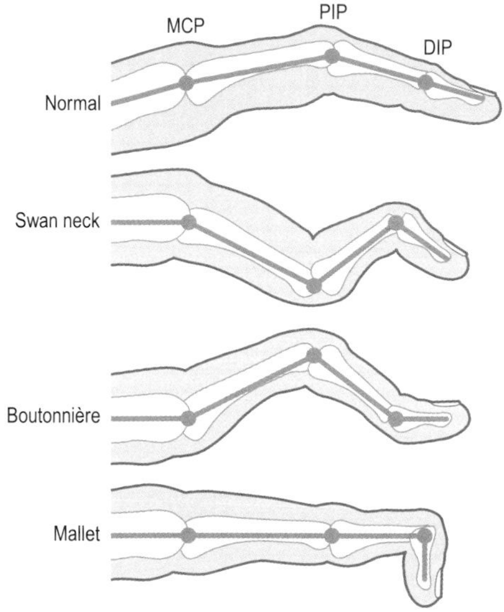

Fig. 5.2 Deformities of the fingers. Swan neck and boutonnière deformities occur in rheumatoid arthritis. Mallet finger occurs with trauma. DIP, distal interphalangeal; MCP, metacarpophalangeal; PIP, proximal interphalangeal.

Q6 Common features of carpal tunnel syndrome

- More common in women
- Unpleasant tingling in the hand
- It may not observe anatomical boundaries, radiating up the arm to the shoulder
- Weakness is uncommon; if it does occur, it affects thumb abduction
- Symptoms are frequently present at night, waking the patient from sleep
- The patient may hang the hand and arm out of bed for relief
- There is thenar muscle wasting (in longstanding cases)
- Commonly associated with pregnancy, diabetes and hypothyroidism

Notes

Q7 Investigations in suspected rheumatoid arthritis (RA)

FBC	Anaemia
U&Es/LFTs	Renal involvement may occur Determine suitability for DMARDs
CRP & ESR	Assess degree of inflammation
CCP	Seropositive RA
X-rays – hands & feet	Joint narrowing, erosions at joint margins
CXR	Rheumatoid lung

Q8 List the extra-articular features of RA

General	Lethargy, malaise, weight loss
Cardiovascular	Pericarditis, pericardial effusion
Respiratory	Nodules, pleural effusion, fibrosing alveolitis, rheumatoid pneumoconiosis (Caplan's syndrome)
Gastrointestinal	Felty's syndrome (splenomegaly + thrombocytopenia)
Neurological	Carpal tunnel syndrome, polyneuropathy, mononeuritis multiplex, atlanto-axial subluxation
Eyes	Scleritis, episcleritis, secondary Sjögren's syndrome
Renal	Amyloidosis, analgesic nephropathy
Skin	Nodules (just below elbow)

Haematological	Anaemia:
	• Microcytic
	  • NSAID induced GI blood loss
	• Normocytic
	  • Chronic disease
	  • Haemolysis
	  • Hypersplenism
	  • Aplastic anaemia (DMARDs)
	• Macrocytic
	  • Drug induced, e.g. methotrexate (folate metabolism)
	  • Associated pernicious anaemia

Vascular	Vasculitis: leg ulcers, nail fold infarcts, gangrene

Notes

Q9 What are the common causes of thoracic spine pain?

Adolescents and young adults	Scheuermann disease Axial spondyloarthritis Disc protrusion (rare)
Middle-aged and elderly	Degenerative change Osteoporotic fracture
Any age	Tumour Infection

Q10 Common causes of low back pain

Cause of low back pain	Features
Degenerative changes in discs and facet joints (spondylosis), e.g. osteoarthritis	Chronic intermittent pain Worse with strenuous activity Stiffness in morning/after immobility May be relieved by gentle activity
Radicular	Pain follows nerve root distribution Symptoms exacerbated by certain movements Usually unilateral
Inflammatory, e.g. ankylosing spondylitis	Insidious onset Worst in the morning/after inactivity Ease with movement Usually young adults Associated extra-articular features (e.g. uveitis)
Trauma, e.g. disc protrusion	Acute onset Usually history of trauma Coughing/straining exacerbates pain May be associated symptoms of root compression

Notes

Q10 Common causes of low back pain

Cause of low back pain	Features
Osteoporotic	Worse with spinal flexion Eased by lying Not usually associated with neurological signs Risk factors for osteoporosis present
Lumbosacral spinal stenosis	Diffuse pain after standing/walking Relieved by spinal flexion
Spinal cord compression	Progressive symptoms of pain – often disturbs sleep Neurological signs May be associated systemic symptoms

Q11 Ankylosing spondylitis

Inflammatory disorder affecting the spine and peripheral joints; part of a spectrum of disorders termed axial spondyloarthritides*	
Incidence	0.5% population Male:female 3:1
Aetiology	Associated with HLA-B27 Environmental factors (e.g. bacteria) have been proposed
Clinical features	Back pain • Classically in early twenties, but <45 years • Insidious onset • Improvement with exercise • No improvement with rest • Pain at night (improves on getting up), marked morning stiffness Pain in one or both buttocks Retention of lumbar lordosis during spinal flexion

Notes

Q11	Ankylosing spondylitis
Other features – think 'As'	Anterior uveitis Inflammation of tendons – Achilles tendonitis Aortic regurgitation and aortitis; A-V heart block Apical lung fibrosis Amyloidosis
Investigations	Inflammatory markers (ESR, CRP) X-rays • Bamboo spine: calcification of intervertebral ligaments and fusion of spinal facet joints • Medial and lateral cortical margins of sacroiliac joints erode and become sclerotic • Inflammatory enthesitis leads to ankylosis and stiffening HLA testing • Rarely performed
Management	Analgesia, NSAIDs Physiotherapy TNF-α blocking drugs when NSAIDs have failed

*Other spondyloarthritides: psoriatic arthritis, reactive arthritis (including Reiter's syndrome), enteropathic arthritis

Notes

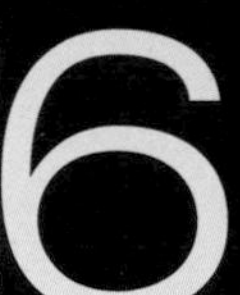

6 The endocrine system

The thyroid exam: common OSCE openers

1. Please examine this patient's neck
2. This patient has noticed a lump in their neck; please examine them
3. Please examine this patient's thyroid status

The thyroid exam: point by point

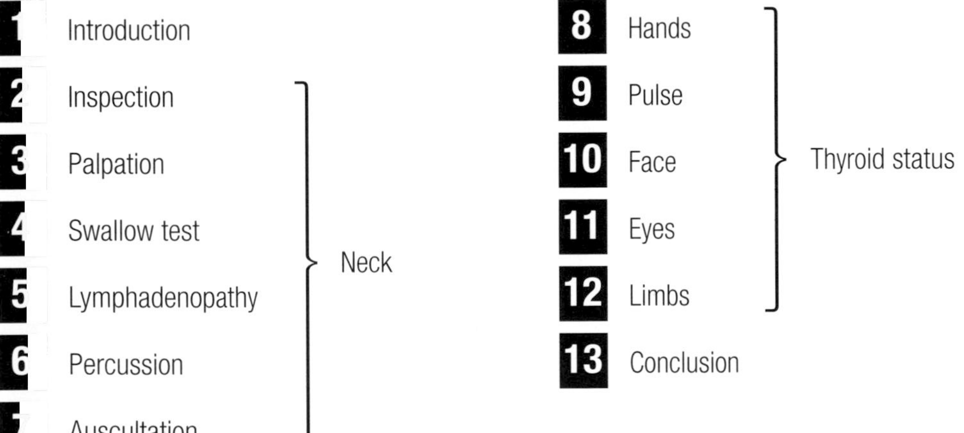

In an exam you may be asked to examine either the neck and/or the thyroid status. Be prepared to perform both examinations.

The thyroid exam: point by point in action

	DO	THINK!	EXAM TIPS
	• Wash hands, introduce yourself • Confirm name/DOB • Position patient sitting in a chair so that you can move behind them	• Immediately start to assess patient's general appearance • Thin, sweaty, flushed (hyper) • Obese, hair loss, dry skin (hypo)	• 80% of patients with a goitre are euthyroid, 10% hyperthyroid and 10% hypothyroid
	• Inspect neck from front and side • Ask patient to slightly extend neck • Ask patient to stick out tongue	• Observe asymmetry or scars • Define location of any swelling • Thyroglossal cyst moves upwards with tongue protrusion	• Goitres are more apparent when the neck is extended as the thyroid and trachea rise
	• Check for pain • Stand behind patient • Palpate thyroid by placing hands on front of neck with index fingers just touching	• Describe approximate size • Shape: diffuse swelling (Graves' disease), uni-nodular or multi-nodular • Consistency: normally soft, hard node(s) suggests carcinoma • Pain: diffuse tenderness (thyroiditis) or localised tenderness (bleeding into cyst) • Mobility: immobility due to fixation to surrounding structures suggests carcinoma • Thrill: thyrotoxicosis	• Patient's neck should be slightly flexed during palpation to relax sternocleidomastoid (SCM) muscles **Q1** What is the differential diagnosis for a neck lump? **Q2** What is the differential diagnosis for a goitre?
	• Ask patient to swallow sips of water while palpating neck	• Thyroid rises with swallowing	• Ask patient to take a sip of water and hold in mouth before swallowing until you are ready to palpate neck
	• Palpate cervical lymph nodes	• Associated cervical lymphadenopathy increases the likelihood of thyroid malignancy	
	• Percuss manubrium to assess for retrosternal extension of goitre		• Although often performed, this is not a reliable test
	• Auscultate over each lobe for a bruit	• Thyroid bruit (+/− thrill) indicates increased blood flow most commonly associated with Graves' disease	• Differential for a thyroid bruit includes a carotid bruit (louder along line of artery)

The thyroid exam: point by point in action

	DO	THINK!	EXAM TIPS

8	• Inspect hands and nails
	• Assess for tremor with paper over outstretched hands
		• Hyperthyroid:
		  • Hot, sweaty, tremulous
		  • Thyroid acropachy (clubbing)
		  • Onycholysis
		  • Palmar erythema
		• Hypothyroid:
		  • Cool and dry
		  • Swelling of skin
			• Acropachy is associated with autoimmune thyroid disease. It is characterised by soft tissue swelling of hands and periosteal hypertrophy (clubbing). It may be associated with pretibial myxoedema and thyroid eye disease

9	• Check pulse	• Hyperthyroid: tachycardia, atrial fibrillation • Hypothyroid: bradycardia	• In hyperthyroidism a mid-diastolic cardiac flow murmur may be present due to increased cardiac output

10	• Observe facial features	• Hyperthyroid:
		  • Flushed, sweaty
		• Hypothyroid:
		  • Coarse facies
		  • 'Peaches and cream' complexion
		  • Loss of outer ⅓ eyebrows
		  • Periorbital puffiness
			Q3 What are the causes of hyperthyroidism?
			Q4 What are the causes of hypothyroidism?

11	• Inspect eyes • Examine eye movements • Assess for lid lag	• Hyperthyroidism (any cause) is associated with lid retraction and lid lag • Graves' disease is associated with exophthalmos and ophthalmoplegia • Lid lag means delay between movement of eyeball and descent of upper eyelid, exposing the sclera above the iris	• Lid retraction is caused by widening of palpebral fissure and is present when white sclera is visible above the iris in the primary gaze position • Graves' ophthalmopathy is typically associated with restriction of upgaze. It is caused by inflammatory infiltration of soft tissues and extraocular muscles

12	• Inspect limbs for pre-tibial myxoedema
	• Assess proximal muscle power (stand from chair without using arms)
	• Assess ankle reflexes
		• Hyperthyroidism:
		  • Pre-tibial myxoedema (Graves') and proximal myopathy
		  • Brisk reflexes
		• Hypothyroidism:
		  • Slow-relaxing reflexes
		  • Non-pitting oedema
			• Carpal tunnel syndrome is associated with hypothyroidism; could consider Phalen's test (see page 71)

13	• To complete my exam I would check thyroid function tests (TFTs) and request an USS neck +/− FNA • Thank patient • Wash hands	• Always finish with a concluding statement to clearly indicate completion of the exam.	

Classic OSCE questions

Q1 Causes of a neck lump

Midline	Goitre (moves up on swallowing) Thyroglossal cyst (moves up on poking out tongue) Submental lymph nodes
Anterior triangle	Lymph nodes Submandibular gland swelling Branchial cyst (anterior to sternocleidomastoid [SCM]) Carotid body tumour Thyroid lobe swelling
Posterior triangle	Lymph nodes
Pre-auricular	Parotid lumps Lymph nodes
Post-auricular	Lymph nodes

Q2 Causes of a goitre

Diffuse	Physiological (puberty, pregnancy) Graves' disease Thyroiditis (Hashimoto's, subacute) Iodine deficiency Drugs (lithium)
Nodular	Multinodular Solitary nodule (adenoma, carcinoma) Fibrotic (Riedel's thyroiditis)
Other	TB Sarcoid Lymphoma

Notes

Q3 Causes of hyperthyroidism

Common	Graves' disease Toxic multinodular goitre Toxic nodule (adenoma)
Less common	Thyroiditis (Hashimoto's, subacute) • May initially be associated with secretion of excess hormone but usually progresses to gland dysfunction and hypothyroidism Drugs (amiodarone) TSHoma Postpartum thyroiditis Ingestion of excess thyroid hormone

Notes

Q4 Causes of hypothyroidism

Primary	Autoimmune thyroiditis • Primary atrophic thyroiditis (no goitre) • Hashimoto's thyroiditis (with goitre) Postpartum thyroiditis Iatrogenic • Post thyroidectomy, radioactive iodine • Drugs (carbimazole, lithium, amiodarone) Iodine deficiency Congenital hypothyroidism
Secondary	Hypothalamic or pituitary disease

The Cushing's exam: common OSCE openers

1. This patient has noticed a change in their appearance; please examine them
2. This patient has noticed an increase in their weight; please examine them

The Cushing's exam: point by point

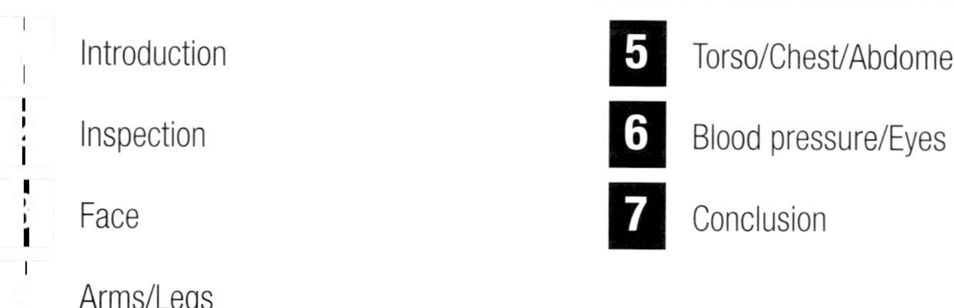

1. Introduction
2. Inspection
3. Face
4. Arms/Legs
5. Torso/Chest/Abdomen
6. Blood pressure/Eyes
7. Conclusion

The Cushing's exam: point by point in action

	DO	THINK!	EXAM TIPS
1	• Wash hands, introduce yourself • Confirm name/DOB • Position patient at 45°	• Immediately start to assess patient's general appearance	
2	• General inspection	• Central obesity • Proximal muscle wasting • Skin striae and bruising	• Patient's skin will be thin and so may have multiple bruises • May be signs of poor wound healing
3	• Examine face	• Round, plethoric, moon face • Acne • Hirsutism • Greasy skin	• May be appropriate to ask patient if they have noticed a change in their appearance • Skin pigmentation occurs with ACTH-dependent cases (Cushing's disease)
4	• Examine arms/legs	• Bruising • Test power of shoulder abduction • Ask patient to stand from chair with arms crossed • Peripheral oedema	• Proximal myopathy characteristic
5	• Examine torso/chest/abdomen	• Supraclavicular fat pads • Interscapular fat pad (buffalo hump) • Kyphosis • Central obesity • Bruising	• Patient may have vertebral wedge fractures due to osteoporosis, leading to kyphosis • Renal transplant scars may be present (long-term steroids may have led to Cushing's)

The Cushing's exam: point by point in action			
	DO	**THINK!**	**EXAM TIPS**
6	• Measure blood pressure • Perform ophthalmoscopy	• Hypertension • Cataracts and hypertensive retinal changes	**Q5** What are the adrenal causes of endocrine hypertension?
7	• To complete my exam, I would check blood sugar, U&Es (hypokalaemia) and urine for glucose	• Always finish with a concluding statement to clearly indicate completion of the exam.	• Consider bone scan for osteoporosis

Classic OSCE questions

Q5 Adrenal causes of endocrine hypertension

Condition	Hormone produced in excess	Associated features
Conn syndrome	Aldosterone	Hypokalaemia
Cushing syndrome	Cortisol	Central obesity, proximal myopathy, fragility fractures, spontaneous bruising, skin thinning, violaceous striae, hypokalaemia
Phaeochromocytoma	Noradrenaline (norepinephrine), adrenaline (epinephrine)	Paroxysmal symptoms, including hypertension, palpitations, sweating

The diabetic foot: common OSCE openers

1. This patient presents with difficulty walking; please examine their feet
2. This patient has pain in his lower limbs; please examine their feet

The diabetic foot exam: point by point

1 Introduction

2 Inspection

3 Temperature

4 Pulses

5 Sensation

6 Reflexes

7 Conclusion

The diabetic foot exam: point by point in action			
	DO	**THINK!**	**EXAM TIPS**
1	• Wash hands, introduce yourself • Confirm name/DOB	• Ensure patient's feet and lower limbs are adequately exposed • Maintain dignity	• Look for clues at bedside, e.g. blood glucose monitor • Look for signs of diabetic complications, e.g. mobility or visual aids

2	• Inspect:
	  • Lower limbs
	  • Feet
	  • Nails
	• Ask patient to stand
	  • Observe foot arch
	  • Observe deformities
		• Skin: infection, acanthosis nigricans (insulin resistance), necrobiosis lipoidica
		• Hair loss on legs/feet
		• Ulcers
		• Cracks/fissures in skin
		• Fungal nail infection
		• Callus formation (abnormal load bearing)
		• Colour of foot: distal pallor = early ischaemia, purple/black = gangrene
		• Joint deformities: claw/hammer toes, prominent metatarsal heads, Charcot's joint
		• Muscle wasting
			Q6 Describe the pathophysiology of diabetic foot ulcers
			Q7a Describe the features of a Charcot joint
			Q7b What are the causes of a Charcot joint?

3	• Check temperature	• Cool feet indicate arterial insufficiency (peripheral vascular disease) • Warm feet occur with neuropathy	• It is not necessary to formally check temperature
4	• Check peripheral pulses (posterior tibial and dorsalis pedis)	• Reduced/absent peripheral pulses indicate arterial insufficiency	• Peripheral pulses can be difficult to palpate

5	• Check sensation using:
	  • Sensory monofilament (pain sensation)
	  • Tuning fork (vibration sense)
		• Sensory loss usually occurs in a stocking distribution. If present, check upper limbs for sensory loss in glove distribution
		• Loss of vibration sense indicates peripheral neuropathy
			• For the causes of peripheral neuropathy see page 41

6	• Test ankle jerks	• Loss of ankle jerks occur in peripheral neuropathy	
7	• Thank patient • Allow to dress	• Discuss results with patient • Arrange further investigations as appropriate	**Q8** Describe further tests/investigations you would like to perform

Classic OSCE questions

Q6 Pathophysiology of diabetic foot ulcers

Ulcer formation is multifactorial due to peripheral and autonomic neuropathy and arterial insufficiency (peripheral vascular disease).

Q7a Features of Charcot (neuropathic) joints

- Joint dislocation
- Pathologic fracture
- Debilitating deformity
- Acute inflammation

Note: often presents acutely as a red, swollen foot which can be difficult to distinguish from infection

Q7b Causes of Charcot joints

- Diabetic neuropathy
- Syphilis
- Chronic alcoholism
- Spinal cord injury
- Syringomyelia
- Cerebral palsy
- Renal dialysis
- (Rheumatoid arthritis)

Q8 Describe further tests/investigations you would like to perform in a patient with diabetic foot disease?

Examine for other microvascular complications:

- Fundoscopy: diabetic retinopathy
- Urinalysis for ketones & microalbuminuria: diabetic nephropathy (also check U&Es)

Check:

- HbA1c: indicates glycaemic control over last 3 months
- Lipid profile: aids assessment of cardiovascular risk
- TFTs: hypothyroidism is associated
- BP & postural BP: assesses cardiovascular risk. Postural hypotension indicates autonomic neuropathy.

Notes

7

The reproductive system

The pregnant abdomen: common OSCE openers

1. Please examine this pregnant woman's abdomen

The pregnant abdomen: point by point

1. Introduction
2. Inspection
3. Blood pressure
4. Palpation
5. Measure symphysial fundal height (SFH)
6. Auscultation
7. Legs
8. Conclusion

The pregnant abdomen exam: point by point in action

	DO	THINK!	EXAM TIPS
1	• Wash hands, introduce yourself • Confirm name/DOB • Position patient semi-recumbent • Expose abdomen from symphysis pubis to xiphisternum	• In late pregnancy examine in left lateral position to avoid vena caval compression (hypotension for mother, hypoxia for fetus)	• Before examining patient, ask her to empty bladder (check urinalysis)
2	• Inspect general demeanour • Look for signs of pregnancy	• Does she appear in pain or distressed? • Cutaneous signs of pregnancy: linea nigra, striae gravidarum (stretch marks), umbilical inversion, dilated superficial veins • Scars: Pfannenstiel (C-section), laparotomy	• It may be possible to see fetal movements (from approximately 24 weeks)
3	• Measure blood pressure	• Patient may have essential hypertension or pregnancy-induced hypertension	

4	• Palpate uterus
	• Ask patient to report any tenderness and watch patient's face throughout
	• Face the woman's head:
	  • Place hands on either side of fundus and palpate fetal parts
	  • With right hand on woman's left side, feel down both sides
	• Face the woman's feet:
	  • With left hand on woman's left side, feel lower part of uterus to identify presenting part
	  • Palpate head gently between fingers
	• Assess fetal lie and presentation and engagement of head in pelvis
		• Palpate lightly to avoid triggering myometrial contraction (makes fetal parts difficult to feel)
		• Estimate liquor volume
		• If fetal parts only palpable on deep palpation this implies large amounts of fluid
		• As palpating down sides of uterus, the side that feels fuller suggests the location of fetal back
		• The lie may be longitudinal (cephalic or breech presentation), oblique or transverse
			• Abdominal organs are displaced during pregnancy
			• Kidneys and liver cannot normally be palpated
			• Bowel sounds may be difficult to hear in late pregnancy
			• From 36 weeks an oblique or transverse lie is abnormal and requires further investigation or treatment

5	• Measure the SFH in centimetres (after 20 weeks)	• At 20 weeks the uterine fundus is at the umbilicus • At 36 weeks the uterine fundus is at the xiphisternum	• After 25 weeks' gestation, a difference of 3 or more between number of weeks of pregnancy and SFH may suggest the baby is small or large for dates. Investigate by ultrasound scan (USS)

	The pregnant abdomen exam: point by point in action		
	DO	**THINK!**	**EXAM TIPS**
6	• Auscultate fetal heart	• From 28 weeks use a Pinard stethoscope over anterior shoulder of fetus • Doppler can be used from 14 weeks	• Percussion of the pregnant abdomen is unnecessary
7	• Examine for peripheral oedema	• May indicate pre-eclampsia	**Q1** What is pre-eclampsia?
8	• To complete my exam I would examine the cardiovascular and respiratory systems and perform a urinalysis	• USS and cardiotocography (CTG) would be performed if any concern	

Classic OSCE questions

Q1	**Pre-eclampsia**
Definition	Disorder of pregnancy associated with hypertension, proteinuria and placental compromise. It is associated with significant maternal and fetal morbidity. Untreated it may result in convulsions (eclampsia)
Risk factors	Obesity Pre-existing hypertension Diabetes Older age First pregnancy
Diagnostic criteria	Hypertension (>140 SBP, >90 DBP) Proteinuria (>0.3 g in 24 hours)
Symptoms	Often asymptomatic Some develop headache and rapidly worsening oedema. There may be a history of upper abdominal pain
Examination	Routine antenatal assessment Include checking for ankle clonus and hyper-reflexia
Treatment	Definitive treatment is delivery of baby Control hypertension

Notes

The breast exam: common OSCE openers

1. This patient is concerned about a breast lump; please examine them

The breast exam: point by point

1. Introduction
2. Inspection
3. Inspection – manoeuvres
4. Palpate breast
5. Palpate nipple
6. Lymph nodes
7. Conclusion

The breast exam: point by point in action			
	DO	**THINK!**	**EXAM TIPS**
1	• Wash hands, introduce yourself and the chaperone • Confirm name/DOB • Ask patient to undress to waist • Sit upright on a chair or bed	• Always offer a chaperone • Male doctors should always have a chaperone	• Be professional • Use your full name

2	• Inspect breasts with patient resting hands on thighs and pectoral muscles relaxed	• Asymmetry?
		• Skin changes:
		  • Skin dimpling occurs where skin remains mobile over underlying cancer
		  • Indrawing of skin where skin is fixed to the cancer
		  • Peau d'orange where the skin looks like orange peel caused by lymphoedema of the breast with swelling between hair follicles
		  • Eczema of nipple/areola may be part of skin disorder, Paget's disease of the nipple or intraductal carcinoma
		• Nipple changes
		  • Nipple inversion is common and often benign. May be malignant (usually asymmetrical)
		  • Small amount of fluid may be discharged by massaging breast. Investigate if persistent or blood-stained
			Q1 What is the differential diagnosis of a breast lump?
			Q2 What are the causes of gynaecomastia?

The breast exam: point by point in action

	DO	THINK!	EXAM TIPS
		• Galactorrhoea common post breastfeeding or caused by drugs, rarely hyperprolactinaemia • Scars from previous surgery (mastectomy, lumpectomy)	
3	• Ask patient to press hands on hips to contract pectoral muscles • Ask patient to raise arms above head • With arms raised above head, ask patient to lean forward to expose whole breast	• Continue to examine for abnormalities described above in these different positions which may exacerbate skin dimpling and accentuate swellings	
4	• Ask patient to lie on bed with hand under head on side to be examined • Check if patient in any pain • Palpate breast tissue	• Think of the breast as a clock face • Palpate each 'hour' from the periphery to the nipple • Compare side for side • Elevate breast to uncover dimpling • Define characteristics of any mass	• If a mass is found, hold between thumb and forefinger. Ask patient to contract pectoral muscles by pushing hands on hips. Note whether mass moves with muscle. Fixation to muscle suggests malignancy
5	• Palpate nipple	• Gently hold between index finger and thumb • Massage breast towards nipple to uncover any discharge	• Test any discharge for blood using urine-testing sticks
6	• Palpate regional lymph nodes	• Palpate axillary lymph nodes • Examine supraclavicular fossa • Palpate cervical lymph nodes	• Assess any palpable masses for size, consistency and fixation
7	• Thank patient • Wash hands	• If lump identified this will need further investigation by imaging and fine needle aspiration	

Classic OSCE questions

Q1 Causes of a breast lump	
Common	Fibroadenoma Fibrocystic breast Abscess Invasive breast cancer Ductal carcinoma in situ
Uncommon	Trauma, fat necrosis Granulomatous mastitis Other cysts (e.g. galactocele)

Notes

Q2 Causes of gynaecomastia

Drugs	Cimetidine Spironolactone Digoxin Antiandrogens (finasteride, bicalutamide) Ketoconazole Methadone
Decreased androgen production	Klinefelter's syndrome
Increased oestrogen levels	Liver cirrhosis Graves' disease Some adrenal tumours
Physiological	Newborn infants of both sexes may show breast development Adolescent gynaecomastia may occur between ages 10–12 but should resolve within 18 months
Unknown	Cause remains unknown in 25%

Notes

The female and male genitalia exams: common OSCE openers

You may be asked to perform an examination of the female or male genitalia using a mannikin in an OSCE. Knowing how to do this sensitively but competently and professionally is an important prerequisite of being a doctor.

The vaginal exam: point by point

1. Introduction
2. Inspection
3. Bimanual examination
4. Speculum examination
5. Cervical smear test
6. Conclusion

The vaginal exam: point by point in action

	DO	THINK!	EXAM TIPS
1	• Introduce yourself and the chaperone • Wash hands and apply gloves • Ask patient to empty bladder first • Ask patient to remove clothes from waist down and position patient appropriately on bed • Provide sheet for patient to cover their lower half • Explain purpose and process of exam	• Warn patient that the exam may be uncomfortable • Maintain patient's dignity	• Be professional • Use your full name

2	• Inspect perineum
	• Ask patient to cough while you examine for prolapse/ incontinence
		• Assess for:
		  • Hair distribution (may be infestation)
		  • Atrophic change (post menopause)
		  • Skin abnormalities
		  • Discharge
		  • Swelling of vulva (e.g. Bartholin glands, cysts)
		  • Ulcers (herpes)
		  • Clitoromegaly (hyperandrogenism)
			Q1 What are Bartholin's glands?
			Q2 What are the causes of vulval skin abnormalities?
			Q3 What are the causes of vaginal discharge?

3	• Bimanual examination (Fig. 7.1) • Lubricate right index/middle finger • Gently insert them into vagina and feel for firm cervix • Push fingers into posterior fornix and lift uterus while pushing abdomen with left hand, palpate uterus between both hands. • Move vaginal fingers to anterior fornix and palpate anterior uterine surface. • Move fingers to lateral fornix and, with your left hand above and lateral to umbilicus, palpate adnexal masses between fingers	• Vulval abnormalities: skin disease, herpes, thrush, malignancy • Cervical abnormalities: polyps or malignancy may be associated with bleeding or ulceration • Tender nodules in posterior fornix suggests endometriosis • Cervical excitation (acute pain on touching cervix): infection, cyst accident or tubal rupture • Fibroids cause uterine irregularity and enlargement	• The normal uterus should feel regular, mobile and the size of a plum • The ovaries are only palpable in very slim patients. Fallopian tubes are not palpable • The uterus is usually anteverted and you will feel its firmness anterior to the cervix. In 15% of patients, the uterus is retroverted and you feel firmness posterior to the cervix (Fig. 7.2) • A large midline mass may be uterine or ovarian. Push the mass upwards with your left hand and feel the cervix with your right hand. If it moves without the cervix, this suggests ovarian pathology

The vaginal exam: point by point in action

	DO	THINK!	EXAM TIPS
	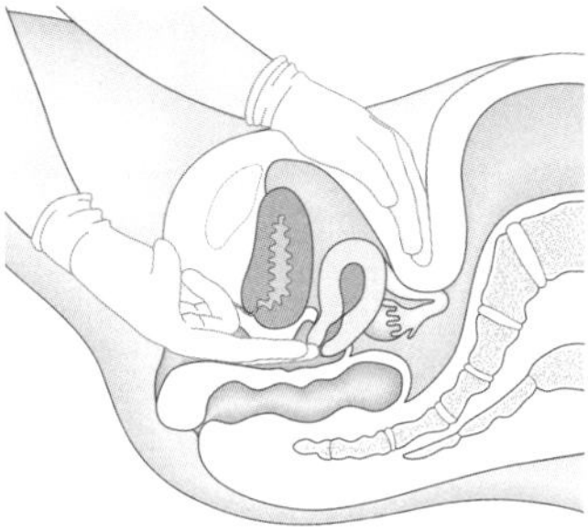 **Fig. 7.1 Bimanual examination of the uterus.** Use your vaginal fingers to push the cervix back and upwards, and feel the fundus with your abdominal hand.	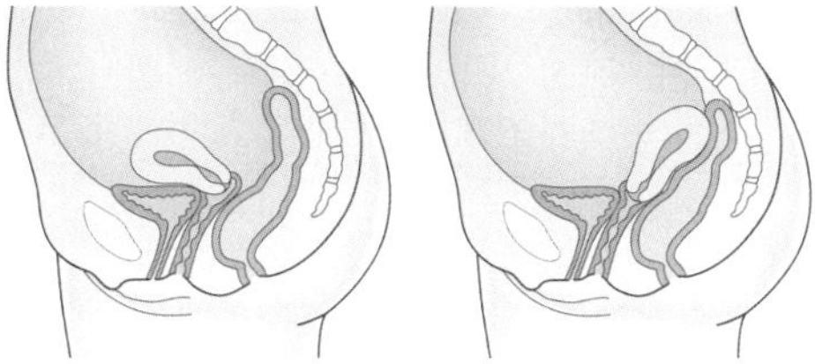 **Fig. 7.2 Coronal section. A** Anteverted uterus. **B** Retroverted uterus.	

4	• Speculum examination
	  • Gently part labia with left hand
	  • Insert lubricated speculum with blades vertical, then rotate through 90° so handles point anteriorly and blades horizontally
	  • Open blades to visualise cervix between them
		• A metal speculum is cold so run under warm water
		• Inspect vaginal or cervical abnormalities (e.g. ulcers, swellings, erosions)
		• Note any discharge
			• If you cannot see cervix, reinsert speculum at a more downward angle as it may lie behind posterior blade

5	• Cervical smear test
	• If already discussed with patient and consent gained then carry out cervical smear test
		• Ensure entire cervix can be visualised with speculum first
		• Two methods:
		  • Liquid-based cytology:
		    • Insert centre of plastic broom into cervical os
		    • Rotate 5 times through 360°
		    • Push broom 10 times against bottom of container
		    • Twirl five times through 360°
		  • Conventional smear:
		    • Insert long blade of spatula into cervical os
		    • Rotate through 360°
		    • Spread once across glass slide
		    • Place slide into fixative for 3 minutes
		    • Remove and leave to dry
			• Liquid-based cytology is the method used in the UK due to improved sensitivity and specificity

6	• Thank patient • Wash hands	• Allow to dress in private	

Classic OSCE questions

Q1 Bartholin's glands

What are they?	Two pea-sized alveolar glands located posterior to the left and right of the vagina
Function	Secrete mucous to lubricate the vagina
Pathology	May become blocked and inflamed resulting in pain (Bartholin's cysts) May then become infected and form an abscess Adenocarcinoma rare

Q2 Causes of vulval skin abnormalities

Dermatitis	Atopic, seborrhoeic, secondary to contact irritant; itchy and erythematous
Psoriasis	Itchy, scaly plaques. Examine elsewhere for plaques
Candidiasis	Itchy, white discharge, dyspareunia, dysuria
Lichen simplex chronicus	Chronic eczematous irritation, thickening and hypertrophy of skin, itchy and erythematous, mucosa not involved
Lichen sclerosus	Chronic whitened plaques in vulva and peri-anal region, hourglass appearance involving perianal skin, loss of labial/ clitoral architecture Itchy
Lichen planus	Itchy, painful erythematous patches Oral/gingival involvement possible
Vulval cancer	Itchy, discharge, bleeding, pain

Notes

Q3 Causes of vaginal discharge	
Physiological	Thick, white, not itchy
Menstruation, miscarriage, cancer	Blood
Candida albicans	Thick, white, itchy, 'cottage cheese' discharge
Bacterial vaginosis (*Gardnerella vaginalis*)	Thin, grey/green, fishy odour, not itchy
Trichomonas	Yellow/green, frothy, itchy, fishy odour
Gonorrhoea	Thick, white/yellow, dysuria, pelvic pain

Notes

The testicular exam: point by point

1. Introduction
2. Inspection
3. Examine penis
4. Examine scrotum and testes
5. Conclusion

The testicular exam: point by point in action

	DO	THINK!	EXAM TIPS
1	• Introduce yourself and a chaperone • Wash hands and apply gloves • Ask patient to expose area from lower abdomen to thighs • Explain purpose and process of exam	• Ensure privacy • Examine patient standing up, unless examining inguinoscrotal area in which case lie patient down	• Be professional • Use your full name
2	• Inspect groin, skin creases, perineum and scrotal skin	• Note hair distribution (may be infestation) • Look for erythema, ulcers, swelling • Scrotal oedema may be caused by local problem (lymphoedema due to pelvic lymphadenopathy) or systemic problem (e.g. heart or liver failure, nephrotic syndrome)	• Patients who shave pubic hair may have dermatitis or folliculitis
3	• Examine penis shaft and position of urethral opening • Retract prepuce and inspect glans for red patches or vesicles	• Hypospadias: urethral opening part way along the penis shaft	• Always draw foreskin forward after examination to prevent paraphimosis • Uniform pearly penile papules around the corona of the glans are normal
4	• Examine scrotum with man standing. Then ask him to lie down if you find a swelling you cannot get above. • Palpate the scrotum and localise both testes • Check size and consistency of each testis • Palpate spermatic cord. Gently pull testis downward and place fingers behind the neck of the scrotum. Feel the spermatic cord and within it the vas • Palpate epididymis • Palpate any swelling and identify whether it arises from scrotum or inguinal canal • Check any inguinoscrotal swelling for a cough impulse	• If both testes are not palpable in scrotum, examine inguinal canal and perineum looking for undescended or ectopic testes • Transilluminate any scrotal swelling with a torch	• A normal testis is approximately 5 cm long • The normal epididymis is only readily felt at the top of the testis • It is possible to 'get above' a true scrotal swelling • If the swelling is caused by an inguinal hernia that has descended into the scrotum, it is impossible to get above it **Q1** What is the differential diagnosis for a scrotal swelling? **Q2** What is a hydrocele and varicocele? **Q3** Describe testicular tumours
5	• Thank patient • Wash hands	• Allow to dress in private	

Q1 Differential of scrotal swelling

Painful swelling	Torsion of testis Epididymo-orchitis Scrotal abscess Torsion of testicular appendage Trauma (scrotal haematoma)
Painless swelling	Testicular tumour Hydrocele Epididymal cyst Varicocele Inguino-scrotal hernia

Q2 Hydrocele and varicocele

Hydrocele	Collection of fluid between visceral and parietal layers of tunica vaginalis Must exclude a reactive hydrocele secondary to underlying tumour Treatment is conservative or surgical
Varicocele	Abnormal dilatation of veins within the pampiniform plexus Palpable as tortuous mass of veins more prominent when patient standing May be asymptomatic, cause pain and be associated with subfertility 97% on left side due to anatomy of left testicular vein draining into left renal vein Treatment by embolisation or surgery

Notes

Q3 Testicular tumours

Incidence	Rare, <1% of all cancers But most common solid tumours in men aged 15–44 years
Risk factors	Age Caucasian ethnicity Family history Cryptorchidism Abnormal testicular development e.g. Klinefelter's syndrome
Pathophysiology	95% germ-cell • 50% non-seminomatous germ cell tumours (e.g. teratomas) • 45% seminomas 4% lymphomas 1% other
Clinical features	Painless swelling Pain
Investigations	USS, CT Alpha-fetoprotein (AFP) produced in non-seminomatous germ-cell tumours Beta human chorionic gonadotropin (β-HCG) produced by seminomas and teratomas
Treatment	Surgical Chemo/radiotherapy

Notes

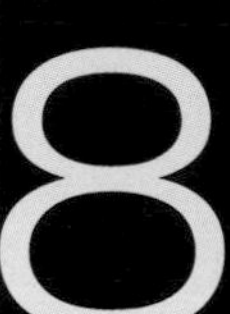

The neonate

The neonatal exam: common OSCE openers

You are unlikely to be asked to perform a neonatal exam during an OSCE but you may be asked to carry this out in the clinical environment. An understanding of the process and abnormalities to look out for is important.

The neonatal exam: point by point

1 Introduction

2 General observation

3 Head

4 Face – eyes, ears, nose, mouth

5 Neck

6 Cardiovascular

7 Respiratory

8 Abdomen

9 Perineum

10 Back

11 Neurological

12 Primitive reflexes

13 Limbs

14 Weight and measurements

15 Conclusion

The neonatal exam: point by point in action

	DO	THINK!	EXAM TIPS

1	• Wash hands, introduce yourself
	• Confirm mother's identity and check baby's wrist bands
	• Explain nature of examination to parents
	• Examine baby in warm environment on firm bed
		• Ask mother:
		  • Maternal history (e.g. diabetes, hereditary illness)
		  • Pregnancy history (e.g. medications)
		  • Birth history (e.g. birthweight, gestation, mode of delivery, prolonged rupture of membranes, Apgar score)
		  • Infants progress (passed meconium and urine?)
			• Term: 37–42 weeks
			• Normal weight: 2500 g
			• Low: <2500 g
			• Very low: <1500 g
			• Extremely low: <1000 g
			Q1 Describe the Apgar score

2	• Observe if baby looks well • Note any dysmorphic features • Observe posture and behaviour • Examine skin • Observe sleepiness • Check temperature	• Skin may look normal, wrinkled or vernix-covered in healthy babies • May be meconium staining • Stork's beak marks on neck, eyelids, glabella due to prominent capillaries will fade with time • Dense capillary haemangiomas (port-wine stains) will not fade. If around the eye suggests Sturge–Weber syndrome	• Erythema toxicum is an idiopathic blanching maculopapular rash affecting face, trunk and limbs – resolves within first few days of birth • Milia (fine white spots) and acne neonatorum (larger cream-coloured spots) are glandular secretions and disappear within 2–4 weeks
3	• Assess baby's head size and shape • Palpate anterior fontanelle • Palpate cranial sutures	• Caput succedaneum is a soft tissue swelling over the vertex due to pressure during labour • Cephalhaematoma is a firm, immobile, parietal swelling caused by local haemorrhage under the cranial periosteum • Subgaleal haemorrhage – boggy, mobile, poorly localised – potentially life threatening • Sunken fontanelle suggests dehydration, bulging suggests raised intracranial pressure (ICP)	• Transient elongation of the head from moulding occurs during vaginal delivery • Abnormal head size requires investigation and imaging

The neonatal exam: point by point in action

	DO	THINK!	EXAM TIPS

4	• Eyes:
	  • Inspect eyes, lids, lashes, eyebrows
	  • Retract lid and check for jaundice
	  • Test ocular movements (doll's eye)
	  • Check for red reflex
	• Ears:
	  • Check size, shape, position
	  • Check external auditory meatus
	• Nose:
	  • Exclude each nostril in turn to ensure baby breathes normally through the other nostril
	• Mouth:
	  • Gently press on lower jaw so baby will open mouth
	  • Examine mouth, tongue, palate
	  • Palpate palate for cleft
	  • Check for tongue tie
		• Yellow crusting without inflammation is common and harmless. Infection causes red eye and purulent secretions
		• Absent red reflex suggests cataract
		• Abnormal ear shape and position may suggest underlying syndrome
		• Glossoptosis: normal sized tongue protruding through small mouth in Down's syndrome
		• Macroglossia: large tongue in Beckwith–Wiedemann syndrome
		• Micrognathia: small jaw associated with cleft palate in Pierre Robin syndrome
			• Teeth usually erupt around 6 months but can be present at birth
			• Cleft palate may involve soft or both hard and soft palates
			• Cleft lip can appear in isolation or in association with it
			• Epstein's pearls are small white mucosal cysts on the palate that disappear spontaneously

5	• Assess neck for asymmetry, sinuses and swellings	• Neck asymmetry is often due to fetal posture • Palpable cervical, axillary, and inguinal regions for lymph nodes which are often present	• Transilluminate any swellings: cystic swellings glow, solid/blood-filled ones do not • A lump in the sternomastoid muscle is caused by a fibrosed haematoma with muscle shortening. May produce torticollis
6	• Observe for pallor, cyanosis, sweat • Palpate apex beat, heaves/thrills • Palpate femoral pulses • Auscultate heart (see Fig. 8.1 for auscultation positions in children)	• Transient murmurs are heard in 2% of neonates, only a minority have a structural heart problem • Heart failure presents with a pale, sweaty baby • Apex beat will be displaced if cardiomegaly, contralateral pneumothorax or effusion present • Weak/absent femoral pulses suggest coarctation	• Do not measure BP in healthy babies • In a term neonate, a normal heart rate is 100–140 beats per minute and respiratory rate is 30–50 breaths per minute • Radio-femoral delay to assess coarctation is not identifiable in the newborn

The neonatal exam: point by point in action

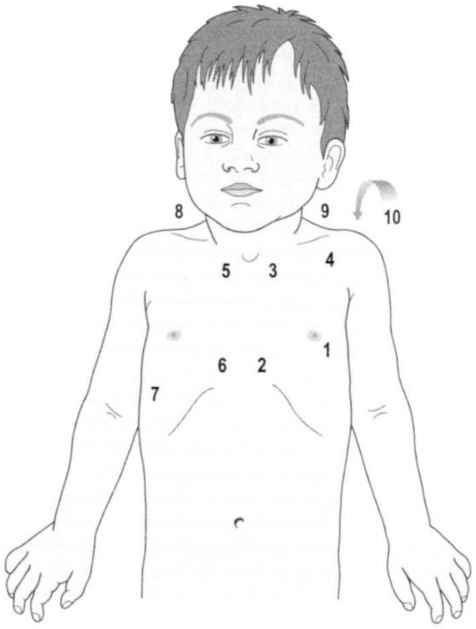

Fig. 8.1 Auscultation positions in infants and children. Recommended order of auscultation: **1,** apex; **2,** left lower sternal edge; **3,** left upper sternal edge; **4,** left infraclavicular; **5,** right upper sternal edge; **6,** right lower sternal edge; **7,** right mid-axillary line; **8,** right side of neck; **9,** left side of neck; **10,** posteriorly.

	DO	THINK!	EXAM TIPS
7	• Observe chest wall/shape • Look for respiratory distress • Count respiratory rate • Auscultate chest anteriorly, laterally and posteriorly	• Signs of respiratory distress include tachypnoea; suprasternal, intercostal and subcostal recession; flaring of nostrils • Causes of respiratory distress: retained lung fluid, infection, immaturity, aspiration, pneumothorax, heart failure, metabolic acidosis	• Breath sounds in the healthy newborn have a bronchial quality compared with older subjects • Percussion of chest not helpful in the newborn
8	• Remove nappy • Inspect abdomen, umbilicus, groin • Palpate abdomen • Check for organomegaly/ masses	• Umbilical hernias are common, easily reduced and complications are rare. Inguinal hernias are common especially in boys • Exomphalos is herniation through the umbilicus containing intestine and other viscera (may be associated with chromosomal abnormalities) • Gastroschisis is a defect in the anterior abdominal wall with intestines herniated through it, without covering membrane	• Abdominal distension from a feed or swallowed air is common • Umbilical cord stump usually separates after 4–5 days • Liver edge and kidneys often palpable in healthy babies • Spleen enlarges down left flank in neonates, not towards right iliac fossa

The neonatal exam: point by point in action

	DO	THINK!	EXAM TIPS

9	• Female:
	  • Abduct legs and gently separate labia for inspection
	• Male:
	  • Inspect shape of penis and check urethral meatus at tip
	  • Palpate testes
	  • Transilluminate any scrotal swelling with a torch
	• Both:
	  • Check anus is patent and normally positioned
		• If testes not palpable, assess for undescended, ectopic or retractile testes
		• Light transmitting through scrotal swelling suggests hydrocele
		• Hypospadias: meatal opening is on ventral aspect of glans, ventral shaft of penis, the scrotum or on the perineum
			• Milky vaginal secretions and vaginal skin tags are normal
			• Slight vaginal bleeding may occur in the first week

10	• Turn baby over • Inspect for pigmented/hairy patches • Inspect curvature • Palpate spine	• Pigmented patches may indicate spina bifida occulta • Hairy, pigmented patches with base that cannot be visualised need further investigation	• Single sacral dimples ($<$5 mm diameter, $<$2.5 cm from anus) with normal skin are common and don't require investigation
11	• Observe symmetry of posture/movement • Look for muscle wasting • Assess tone • Assess power: look for strong symmetrical trunk, limb movements and grasp • Check sensation • Check eyesight	• Movements should be equal on both sides. Tone may be floppy post-feed • Hypotonia may present with 'frog-like' posture with abducted hips and extended elbows (Down's syndrome, meningitis, sepsis) • Sensation should be checked using gentle stimuli. Do not use painful stimuli. • Check eyesight by carrying the alert baby to a dark corner, eyes should open wide. The reverse occurs in bright environments	• Reflexes are brisk in term infants with a few beats of clonus. Plantar reflex usually extensor. Only assess tendon reflexes in babies with neurological problems **Q2** Describe the brachial plexus injuries that may be sustained at birth

12	• Primitive reflexes:
	  • Grasp responses
	  • Ventral suspension
	  • Place and step reflexes
	  • Moro reflex
	  • Root and suck responses
	  • Asymmetric tonic neck reflex
		• Primitive reflexes are lower motor neuron (LMN) responses present at birth but suppressed by 6 months
		• May be absent or asymmetrical if neurological problems
			• Not routinely performed but you should have a knowledge of them

The neonatal exam: point by point in action			
	DO	**THINK!**	**EXAM TIPS**
13	• Inspect limbs and count digits • Observe position of feet • Examine hips	• Talipes equinovarus: foot plantar-flexed and rotated with sole facing medially • Talipes calcaneovalgus: foot dorsiflexed, heel prominent, sole faces laterally • Risk factors for developmental dysplasia of the hips (DDH): family history, breech delivery, positional talipes, oligohydramnios	• Single palmer crease associated with Down's syndrome (can be normal) • Arrange hip USS if concerned about DDH
14	• Weigh baby • Measure head circumference • Measure crown–heel length of baby	• Repeat measurements three times, noting the largest measurement. • Record on centile chart	
15	• Final top-to-toe inspection • Answer any parental questions		

Classic OSCE questions

Q1 Apgar score

Score	0	1	2
Heart rate	Absent	<100 bpm	>100 bpm
Respiratory effort	Absent	Slow, irregular	Good, strong
Muscle tone	Flaccid	Some flexion of arms and legs	Active movement
Reflex irritability	No responses	Grimace	Vigorous crying, sneeze or cough
Colour	Blue, pale	Pink body, blue extremities	Pink all over

Healthy neonates score 8-10 at 1 and 5 minutes

Notes

Q2 Erb's palsy and Klumpke's palsy

	Erb's palsy	Klumpke's palsy
Pathology	Brachial plexus roots C5/C6	Brachial plexus roots C8/T1
Injury	Shoulder dystocia during birth	Breech delivery with excessive traction to arm
Features	'Waiter's tip' position Arm cannot be raised by side Shoulder adducted Arm internally (medially) rotated Forearm extended Elbow extended Failure to extend wrist Sensory loss lateral arm	Sensory loss C8/T1 dermatome (medial forearm and hand) Claw hand Wasting small muscles of hand May be associated with Horner's syndrome due to involvement of T1

Notes

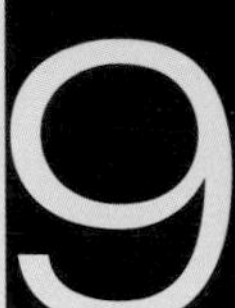

The critically ill patient

Common OSCE openers

Examination of the critically ill patient is a common OSCE scenario through the use of a mannikin. Possible openers include:

1. Please examine this critically ill patient
2. The nurses express concern about this patient's sudden deterioration; please examine them
3. This patient appears very unwell; please examine them and propose a differential diagnosis

Examination of the critically ill patient: point by point

The ABCDE approach provides a standardised framework for simultaneously assessing and treating life-threatening problems in critically ill patients.

1 Initial assessment

2 Call for help

3 Assess the airway (A)

4 Airway manoeuvres (A)

5 Airway adjuncts (A)

6 Assess the breathing (B)

7 Appropriate investigations/interventions (B)

8 Assess the circulation (C)

9 Appropriate investigations/interventions (C)

10 Assess conscious level (D)

11 Assess pupils (D)

12 Check capillary blood glucose (D)

13 Expose and assess patient (E)

14 Check temperature (E)

15 Repeat cycle above

Examination of the critically ill patient: point by point in action

	DO	THINK!	EXAM TIPS
1	• If the patient is conscious: wash hands, introduce yourself, confirm name/DOB • If the patient is unconscious: check pulse/breathing and if in cardiac or respiratory arrest, summon team and begin CPR	• Always ensure your own safety • Use personal protective equipment as appropriate	• The approach to the critically ill patient is time critical • Treat each problem as you meet it and don't move on until resolved
2	• Call for help if not already done so	• Do not delay calling for help	• Even in an exam when you are being assessed, part of the assessment is your recognition of the need for help

3	• If patient is speaking then airway is patent
	• Otherwise:
	  • Look for signs of airway obstruction
	  • Look inside mouth
	  • Listen for abnormal airway noises
	• Administer high flow O_2 via non-rebreather mask at 15 L/minute
		• Signs of airway obstruction: accessory muscle use, supraclavicular or subcostal indrawing, 'seesaw' breathing (chest moves in, abdomen moves out)
		• Foreign objects in mouth: blood, vomit, secretions
		• Consider use of Yankauer suction to remove foreign objects
			• Never forget to apply the O_2 (common mistake when role-playing with a mannikin)
			• Aim O_2 saturations of >94% except in patients at risk of type 2 respiratory failure (e.g. chronic obstructive pulmonary disease [COPD]) where >88% is acceptable
			Q1 Describe different airway noises and possible causes

4	• Open the airway with a head tilt and chin lift or jaw thrust	• Simple manoeuvres can improve the airway until more definitive methods are secured	
5	• Consider use of adjuncts to maintain the airway, e.g. oropharyngeal (Guedel) or nasopharyngeal airways • More definitive airway support (tracheal intubation) will require an anaesthetist	• Measure the size of oropharyngeal airway against the patient's own jaw • Never use a nasopharyngeal airway if base of skull fracture suspected	• Lubricate the nasopharyngeal airway adjunct for ease of insertion • Use of a safety pin prevents migration of proximal end beyond the nasal orifice

Examination of the critically ill patient: point by point in action

	DO	THINK!	EXAM TIPS
6	• Count respiratory rate (RR) • Check oxygen saturations • Assess chest expansion • Palpate trachea • Percuss/auscultate chest	• Normal RR 12–20 breaths/min • >30 breaths/min or <10 breaths/min is a sign of critical illness • Beware situations where pulse oximeter reading is unreliable • Assess for chest wall deformity and chest expansion • Check for subcutaneous emphysema (pneumothorax or trauma) or a flail segment • Trachea deviates towards collapse • Trachea deviates away from effusion/tension pneumothorax • Percuss/auscultate to detect pneumothorax, effusions, consolidation, oedema Consider drug causes when respiratory rate <10 breaths/min (see Chapter 10)	**Q2** In what situations would the pulse oximetry reading be unreliable?
7	• Check arterial blood gas (ABG) • Request portable CXR	• Valuable information about arterial oxygen, carbon dioxide, acid base status	• See Chapter 2 for causes of acid/base abnormalities
8	• Check capillary refill time (CRT) • Skin temperature • Check pulse rate and rhythm • Check central/peripheral pulses • Check blood pressure • Examine jugular venous pressure (JVP) • Auscultate heart	• Normal CRT <2 secs • Delayed CRT: shock • Heart rate (HR) <50 beats/min or >90 beats/min requires further investigation. HR >130 beats/min requires immediate attention • Weak peripheral pulses: hypovolaemia/poor cardiac output • Bounding pulse: sepsis • JVP abnormalities: see page 7	• Generally speaking, if radial pulse is present, systolic blood pressure (SBP) >90 mmHg • If femoral pulse impalpable, SBP <60 mmHg **Q3** How do you identify sepsis? **Q4** Describe the immediate management of sepsis
9	• Obtain IV access (intraosseous [IO] if impossible) • Take full set of bloods and cross match • 12-lead ECG • Monitor fluid balance and consider urinary catheter	• Insert either 14- or 16-gauge cannula (×2 if major haemorrhage) • FBC, U&Es, LFTs, coagulation screen, glucose, cross match • Fluid bolus (250–500 mL crystalloid solution) if hypotensive	• Urinary catheters have an associated morbidity but if patient obtunded or unable to pass urine, insert catheter

Examination of the critically ill patient: point by point in action

	DO	THINK!	EXAM TIPS
10	• Assess conscious level according to AVPU (alert, verbal, pain, unresponsive) or Glasgow Coma Scale (GCS) • Consider naloxone if appropriate (see Chapter 10)	• Any change in conscious level is concerning • Causes of unconsciousness: hypoxia, hypercapnia, cerebral hypoperfusion, hypoglycaemia, sedative medications	• Although now widely used, the GCS was originally validated in patients with traumatic brain injury • The GCS is more sensitive to changes in conscious level **Q5** Describe the AVPU and GCS scale
11	• Examine the pupils for size, symmetry and light reflex	• Symmetrical change in pupil size: drug or metabolic cause (e.g. miosis in opiate toxicity, mydriasis in anticholinergics – see Chapter 10) • Asymmetrical pupils: structural lesion	• A unilateral dilated pupil in a patient with altered conscious level requires urgent investigation (CT)
12	• Check capillary blood glucose	• **ABC D**on't **E**ver **F**orget **G**lucose • Hypoglycaemia (<4 mmol/L) requires immediate treatment with 100 mL 20% dextrose	• Often inappropriately referred to as 'BM' on the ward – appropriate terminology is capillary blood glucose • You should be familiar with how to perform a capillary blood glucose measurement – this may be tested in an OSCE
13	• Examine patient thoroughly	• Examine for evidence of trauma, haemorrhage, rash	• Ensure the patient is adequately exposed (while maintaining dignity)
14	• Measure tympanic (+/− core) temperature	• If hypothermic (<35 °C), confirm on core (rectal) temperature • If hyperthermic (>37.8 °C), take blood cultures and consider antibiotics • Consider drug causes of hyperthermia (see Chapter 10)	• Hypothermia should be treated immediately with a Bair Hugger warming system
15	• Continually repeat the cycle from the top	• Continue to question what further investigations are required, the differential diagnosis and who should be contacted	• Remember not to move on from each point until the problem has been addressed and continually go back to reassess

Classic OSCE questions

Q1 Causes of airway noises

Silent airway	Complete airway obstruction
Stridor	Harsh noise, loudest in inspiration Partial obstruction around the larynx If febrile, consider supraglottitis Otherwise consider foreign bodies, laryngeal trauma, burns, tumours
Snoring	Partial obstruction from soft tissues of mouth and oropharynx
Gurgling	Secretions, blood, vomit in the oropharynx
Grunting	Occurs during expiration and implies respiratory muscle fatigue Improves gas exchange by creating positive end-expiratory pressure to prevent alveolar collapse
Wheeze	When loudest in expiration relates to intrathoracic obstruction of small bronchi and bronchioles, most often in asthma/COPD

Notes

Q2 Unreliable pulse oximetry values

Poor waveform	Hypoperfusion (use ear probe if poor hand perfusion) Hypothermia Rapid irregular pulse (e.g. atrial fibrillation [AF]) Movement artefact
False normal or high reading	Carboxyhaemoglobinaemia (CO poisoning) Methaemoglobinaemia (hereditary or acquired)
False low reading	Nail varnish (remover)/ false fingernails Severe anaemia Skin pigmentation Methaemoglobinaemia

Q3 How do you identify sepsis?

Systemic inflammatory response syndrome (SIRS) criteria

If clinical suspicion of infection and 2 or more of the following criteria are present – THINK SEPSIS

1 Temperature <36 °C or >38 °C
2 Pulse >90 bpm
3 WCC <4 or >12 × 10^9/L
4 RR >20 breaths/min
5 New confusion
6 Blood glucose >7.7 mmol/L (in absence of diabetes)

Q4 Immediate management of sepsis

The Sepsis Six therapeutic bundle (within 1 hour)

1 O_2 to target sats >94% (unless COPD: 88–92%)
2 IV fluids
3 Take blood cultures
4 IV antibiotics
5 Measure lactate and white cell count (WCC)
6 Monitor fluid balance and urine output

Notes

Q5a	**The AVPU scale**
A	Alert
V	Responds to Voice
P	Responds to Pain
U	Unresponsive

Q5b	**The Glasgow Coma Scale**
Eye opening (E)	
4	Spontaneously
3	To speech
2	To pain
1	No response
Best verbal response (V)	
5	Orientated
4	Confused
3	Inappropriate words
2	Inappropriate sounds
1	No verbal response
Best motor response (M)	
6	Obeys commands
5	Localises to painful stimulus
4	Normal flexion
3	Abnormal flexion
2	Extends to painful stimulus
1	No response

Notes

10

The poisoned patient

Common OSCE openers

Although you would never be asked to examine an acutely poisoned patient in an exam, examination of the poisoned patient is a common OSCE scenario through the use of a mannikin. Possible openers include:

1. Please examine this patient
2. This patient has taken an overdose; please examine them to determine what substance may be involved

Examination of the poisoned patient: point by point

1. Initial assessment
2. Call for help
3. Airway
4. Breathing
5. Circulation
6. Conscious level
7. Pupils
8. Capillary blood glucose
9. Temperature
10. Expose and systematic examination
11. Repeat cycle above

The examination described above is similar to that of the critically ill patient described in Chapter 9. The emphasis here, however, is on detecting the abnormalities commonly found in poisoned patients.

Examination of the poisoned patient: point by point in action

	DO	THINK!	EXAM TIPS
1	• If patient is conscious: wash hands, introduce yourself, confirm name/DOB • If patient is unconscious: check pulse/breathing and if in cardiac or respiratory arrest, summon team and begin CPR	• Always ensure your own safety • Use personal protective equipment as appropriate • Patient may have drugs/ needles in personal possession	• Adopt a systematic, stepwise approach to ensure all aspects covered
2	• Call for help if not already done so		• Management of the poisoned patient is complex • Involve senior clinicians at an early stage
3	• Examine for signs of airway obstruction • Administer oxygen as appropriate • Open the airway with maneuvers/adjuncts as appropriate (see Chapter 9 for a full description of airway assessment)	• Consider the presence of foreign objects in the mouth (e.g. drugs, packet) • Signs of ulceration, oedema of oropharynx: consider ingestion of a corrosive substance (acid/ alkali). • Urgent intubation may be required for airway protection	• It may not always be possible to establish precisely what the poison is and so management should follow basic principles of supportive care
4	• Count respiratory rate • Check oxygen saturations • Consider arterial blood gas (ABG) • Consider naloxone if features of opioid toxicity	• Reduced respiratory rate: consider opioid toxidrome • Clinically cyanotic patient with low finger probe saturations but normal/ high pO_2 on ABG with supplemental oxygen: consider methaemoglobinaemia and measure methaemoglobin concentration	**Q1** Describe the different toxidromes and associated drugs
5	• Check pulse rate and rhythm • Check capillary refill time • Check blood pressure • Perform 12-lead ECG • Obtain IV access and take bloods	• Fluid resuscitate if hypotensive • ECG: in particular check QRS and QT duration • Untreated QRS prolongation associated with VT/VF • Untreated QT prolongation associated with torsades de pointes (TdP) • Check paracetamol level at 4 hrs post ingestion or immediately if patient presents >4 hrs after ingestion • Check salicylate level if aspirin ingested	• QT interval inversely proportional to heart rate • Corrected QT interval (QTc) estimates QT at HR of 60 bpm • Normal QTc <440ms (males) and <460ms (females) • QTc >500 ms associated with increased risk of TdP **Q2** What are the common drug causes of QRS/QT prolongation and what would the appropriate treatment be?

Examination of the poisoned patient: point by point in action

	DO	THINK!	EXAM TIPS
6	• Assess Glasgow Coma Scale (GCS)	• Depressed consciousness: sedatives/opioids • Agitation: sympathomimetics, serotonergic agents • Consider naloxone if appropriate (see point 4)	• Flumazenil not recommended for benzodiazepine toxicity due to risk of seizures
7	• Assess pupils	• Miosis: opioids, olanzapine, organophosphorous insecticides • Mydriasis: tricyclic antidepressants, ethanol, amphetamines, antihistamines • Nystagmus: ethanol, amphetamines, benzodiazepines, selective serotonin reuptake inhibitors (SSRIs) • Divergent squint: tricyclic antidepressants	• Pupils can provide many clues to the drug that has been ingested
8	• Check capillary blood glucose	• Hypoglycaemia may be the result of ethanol as well as drug ingestion • Hypoglycaemia (<4 mmol/L) requires immediate treatment with 100 mL 20% dextrose	• **ABC D**on't **E**ver **F**orget **G**lucose
9	• Check tympanic (+/− core) temperature	• Stimulant/serotonergic/anticholinergic drugs associated with hyperthermia • Hyperthermia associated with significant morbidity and mortality	• Critical to reduce temperature urgently through ice packs, external cooling, cooled fluids
10	• Examine patient thoroughly	• Consider specific findings, e.g. needle track marks, clonus (serotonin syndrome) • Consider urine/oral drugs screen	• Clonus is more obvious peripherally, e.g. ankles • In severe cases ocular clonus may be present • Urine/oral drugs screens are helpful but take time to process and so don't help immediate management
11	• Continually repeat from the top	• Narrow the differential as the results of investigations are available	

Classic OSCE questions

Q1 The toxidromes

Toxidrome	Clinical features	Example drugs
Opioid	Depressed consciousness Respiratory depression Miosis Hypotension	Heroin Methadone Morphine Dihydrocodeine
Sedative	Depressed consciousness Ataxia Dysarthria Nystagmus	Ethanol Benzodiazepines GHB/GBL Barbiturates
Sympathomimetic	Hypertension Tachycardia Agitation Hyperreflexia Seizures	Cocaine Amphetamines 'Ecstasy'
Serotonin toxicity (serotonin syndrome)	Neuromuscular hyperactivity (clonus, hypertonia) Autonomic instability (temperature, labile BP) Altered conscious level (agitation, coma)	SSRIs Amphetamines Cocaine Tramadol Novel psychoactive substances
Anticholinergic	Dry mouth, skin Mydriasis Hyperthermia Tachycardia Delirium Urinary retention Ileus	Tricyclic antidepressants (e.g. amitriptyline) Antihistamines (e.g. diphenhydramine) Antipsychotics (e.g. chlorpromazine) Antimuscarinic (e.g. hyoscine)
Cholinergic	Increased sweating/lacrimation Miosis Involuntary defecation/urination Bradycardia Muscle paralysis Respiratory failure	Organophosphorous insecticides Carbamate insecticides Nerve agents
Methaemoglobinaemia	Cyanotic appearance Low finger probe saturations but normal/high pO_2 on ABG with supplemental oxygen Breathlessness Chest pain	Sodium nitrite Amyl nitrite (poppers) Local anaesthetics (e.g. lidocaine, prilocaine) Antibiotics (e.g. trimethoprim, dapsone)

Q2 Common drug causes of QRS/QT prolongation

ECG abnormality	Example drug	Treatment
QRS prolongation	Tricyclic antidepressants Local anaesthetics Quinine sulphate	Sodium bicarbonate
QT prolongation	Antipsychotics SSRIs Methadone	Magnesium sulphate

Notes

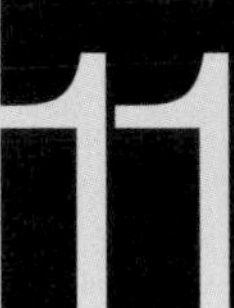

The psychiatric patient

Common OSCE openers

1. This patient has been referred by their GP due to concerns about low mood; please perform a mental state examination
2. This patient has been brought in by the police following a complaint from their partner that they were behaving strangely at home; please talk to them in the next 10 minutes

The mental state examination (MSE): point by point

1 Introduction

2 Appearance/behaviour

3 Speech

4 Emotion

5 Perception

6 Thoughts

7 Insight

8 Cognition

9 Conclusion

A useful pneumonic to remember the above format is ASEPTIC

The mental state examination: point by point in action			
	DO	THINK!	EXAM TIPS
1	• Wash hands, introduce yourself • Confirm name/DOB • Explain purpose and process of interview	• Ensure patient is comfortable • Emphasise you will maintain confidentiality	• Try to develop rapport early, particularly before raising more sensitive topics of discussion

2	• Assess appearance and behaviour	• Consider appearance:
		  • Clothing
		  • Hygiene/grooming
		  • Tattoos or scars (self-harm)
		  • Evidence of relevant physical disease (e.g. thyrotoxicosis)
		  • Evidence of substance misuse (e.g. injection tracks)
		  • Facial expression
		• Consider behaviour
		  • Eye contact
		  • Rapport
		  • Engagement
		  • Level of arousal (calm, agitated)
		  • Abnormal activity (e.g. posturing or involuntary movements)
			• Think of the patient in front of you as a photograph or video that you have to describe to someone who cannot see it
			Q1 Describe the different types of abnormal behaviour

3	• Assess speech	• Consider:
		  • Language used
		  • Tone
		  • Volume
		  • Rate
		  • Fluency
		  • Articulation
			• In this part of the assessment the focus is on the form of speech rather than content
			Q2 Define the different types of abnormal speech

4	• Assess emotion	• Assess the patient's mood and affect
		• Use screening questions to ask about mood:
		  • Have you felt down, sad or hopeless in the last month?
		  • Have you lost interest in things you used to enjoy?
		• Ask about biological symptoms of low mood
			• Mood: a person's emotional experience over time
			• Affect: immediate expression of a person's mood
			• A way of conceptualising this is to consider the relationship between the weather (affect) and the season or climate (mood)
			Q3 What are the biological (physical) symptoms of depression?

The mental state examination: point by point in action

	DO	THINK!	EXAM TIPS
5	• Assess perception	• Abnormal perceptions are assessed via the history and observing the patient's behavior, i.e. apparent responses to hallucinations or unobserved stimuli • It is also useful to use specific screening questions, such as: • Do you ever hear (see/taste/smell) things when there is nobody/nothing else there?	• In mental illness, the ability to distinguish between what is real and not real may become impaired **Q4** Describe the different abnormalities of perception

6	• Assess thoughts (content and form)	• Thought content:
		  • Preoccupations
		  • Ruminations
		  • Abnormal beliefs, e.g. delusions
		• Screening questions:
		  • What has been on your mind recently?
		  • Do you have any thoughts that you can't get out of your head?
		• Thought form:
		  • How are thoughts linked?
		  • Speed and directness of thoughts
		  • Sequencing and abstraction
		• Thought form is largely assessed by observation, unlike thought content which requires specific questions to assess properly
			• Thought content describes themes occupying the patient's mind
			• Thought form describes how the patient thinks (rather than the actual content)
			Q5 Describe the different abnormal beliefs
			Q6 Describe the different thought forms

7	• Assess insight	• Consider:
		  • Recognition that abnormal mental experiences are abnormal
		  • Agreement that these experiences equal to a mental illness
		  • Acceptance of the need for treatment for a mental illness
		• Possible questions:
		  • What do you think is causing this?
		  • Do you think you need any treatment?
			• Remember that insight is a very important part of the mental state examination as without it there will likely be non-compliance with treatment interventions

The mental state examination: point by point in action

	DO	THINK!	EXAM TIPS
8	• Assess cognition	• Core cognitive functions include: • Consciousness • Orientation (time, place) • Memory • Attention/concentration • Intelligence	• If cognitive deficit is suspected, it must be evaluated using a standard test • Shorter screening tools: • Abbreviated Mental Test (AMT) • 4AT • Longer more detailed tools: • Mini-Mental State Examination (MMSE) • Montreal Cognitive Assessment (MoCA)
9	• Conclusion	• Summarise findings and consider a differential diagnosis and management plan • A risk assessment is a crucial part of every psychiatric assessment, pulling together the history, MSE and collateral information	• Don't forget to thank the patient and tell them you will feed back to them once you have considered your findings • It is unlikely you will be asked to perform a risk assessment in an exam but in the clinical setting, you must consider: • Who is at risk? • The nature of the risk • The likelihood of risk **Q7** Describe the main components of a suicide risk assessment **Q8** Describe risk factors for completed suicide

Classic OSCE questions

Q1 Different types of abnormal behaviour

Term	Definition
Agitation	A combination of psychic anxiety and excessive, purposeless motor activity
Compulsion	A stereotyped action that the patient cannot resist performing repeatedly
Disinhibition	Loss of control over normal social behaviour
Motor retardation	Decreased motor activity, usually a combination of fewer and slower movements
Posturing	The maintenance of bizarre gait or limb positions

Q2 Speech abnormalities

Term	Definition
Clang associations	Thoughts connected by having a similar sound rather than by meaning
Mutism	Absence of speech without impaired consciousness
Neologism	An invented word, or a new meaning for an established word
Pressure of speech	Rapid, excessive, continuous speech (due to pressure of thought)
Word salad	Meaningless string of words, often with loss of grammatical construction
Echolalia	Senseless repetition of the interviewer's words

Q3 Biological (physical) symptoms of depression

Appetite and weight changes (usually decreased)
Loss of concentration
Loss of libido
Menstrual irregularities
Unexplained pain
Constipation
Sleep disturbance

Notes

Q4 Abnormalities of perception

Depersonalisation	Subjective experience of feeling unreal Patients find difficult to describe Ask: "Have you ever felt that you were not real?"
Derealisation	Subjective experience that the surrounding environment is unreal Ask: "Have you ever felt that the world around you wasn't real?"
Hallucination	False perception arising without a valid stimulus from the external world Categorised according to sensory modality Usually indicates mental illness, although can occur naturally when falling asleep (hypnagogic) or waking up (hypnopompic)
Illusion	False perception that is an understandable misinterpretation of a real stimulus in the external world Commonly occur among people with impairment of vision or hearing Suggestive of organic illness such as delirium, dementia or alcohol withdrawal
Pseudohallucination	False perception that is perceived as part of the patient's internal experience Occurs within the patient themselves They lack the vividness and reality of true hallucinations Patient not usually distressed

Notes

Q5 Abnormal beliefs: definitions

Term	Definition
Delusion	An abnormal belief, held with total conviction, which is maintained in spite of proof or logical argument to the contrary and is not shared by others from the same culture
Delusional perception	A delusion that arises fully formed from the false interpretation of a real perception, e.g. a traffic light turning green confirms that aliens have landed on the rooftop
Magical thinking	An irrational belief that certain actions and outcomes are linked, often culturally determined by folklore or custom, e.g. fingers crossed for good luck
Overvalued ideas	Beliefs that are held, valued, expressed and acted on beyond the norm for the culture to which the person belongs
Thought broadcasting	The belief that the patient's thoughts are heard by others
Thought insertion	The belief that thoughts are being placed in the patient's head from outside
Thought withdrawal	The belief that thoughts are being removed from the patient's head

Notes

Q6 Thought form: definitions

Term	Definition
Circumstantiality	Trivia and digressions impairing the flow but not direction of thought
Concrete thinking	Inability to think abstractly
Flights of ideas	Rapid shifts from one idea to another, retaining sequencing
Loosening of associations	Logical sequence of ideas impaired. Subtypes include knight's-move thinking, derailment, thought blocking and, in its extreme form, word salad
Perseveration	Inability to shift from one idea to the next
Pressure of thought	Increased rate and quantity of thoughts

Q7 Suicide risk assessment

Ideation (thoughts) should have been elicited as part of main mental state assessment	
Plan	Are the means available or readily accessible? Does the patient know how to use these means? What is the lethality of the plan? What is the likelihood of rescue?
Intent	Have preparations been made? Has an attempt already been made or has the patient practised the suicidal act? What is the strength of the intent? What is the accessibility of support systems including psychiatric follow-up? What are the stressors that threaten the patient's ability to cope?

Notes

Q8 Risk factors for suicide

Risk factors	Protective factors
Previous history of suicide attempts Family history of suicide Co-existing mental illness History of childhood abuse or other adverse experiences History of alcohol or substance misuse Impulsive or aggressive tendencies Loss (social, relationship, work, financial) Isolation Access to lethal methods	Effective treatment for physical, mental illness Family or other support Cultural or religious beliefs against suicide

Notes

12

Classic OSCE cases

Parkinson's disease: common OSCE openers

1. This patient has noticed loss of facial expression and tremor; please examine them
2. This patient has noticed a deterioration in their hand writing; please examine them
3. This patient has been dizzy and falling over; please examine them

The Parkinson's exam: point by point

1. Introduction
2. General inspection
3. Assess speech
4. **T**remor
5. **R**igidity
6. **A**kinesia
7. **P**ostural instability (gait)
8. Glabellar tap
9. Writing
10. Function
11. Parkinson-plus syndrome
12. Conclusion

Remember the pneumonic 'TRAP' for the examination sequence in Parkinson's disease.

The Parkinson's exam: point by point in action

	DO	THINK!	EXAM TIPS
1	• Wash hands, introduce yourself • Check patient not in pain	• Ensure patient adequately exposed • Maintain dignity	• Be professional • Use your full name
2	• Observe patient from the end of the bed	• Hypomimia ('mask-like' face) • Drooling	• Be courteous • Explain to the patient what you are doing • Look for walking aids
3	• Ask patient to confirm name/DOB	• Speech will be slow, monotonous • Hypophonia (quiet) • Minimal facial movements	• Points 1–3 can be done almost simultaneously
4	• Observe tremor with hands resting on pillow/knee • Assess effect of posture by asking patient to hold hands out	• 3–5 Hz, coarse 'pill-rolling' tremor • Improves with posture	• Resting tremor is hallmark of Parkinson's disease • Consider other causes of tremor (see page 46)
5	• Assess for rigidity • Take hand and support elbow • Flex/extend wrist and elbow • Ask patient to move contralateral arm up and down	• Lead pipe rigidity is present in parkinsonism • 'Cog-wheeling' occurs when tremor is superimposed on rigidity	• Ask patient to move contralateral arm up and down: augments hypertonia
6	• Ask patient to 'play the piano' • Touch thumb to each finger in turn	• Look for bradykinesia	**Q1** What are the causes of parkinsonism? **Q2** What are the treatments used in Parkinson's disease?
7	• Ask patient to walk across the room, turn 180° and return	• Difficulty initiating and stopping • Festinant, shuffling gait • Lack of arm swing • Unsteady with propulsion/retropulsion (tendency to fall forwards/backwards)	• Observe patient turning 180° • Most people will do this with 2–3 steps. People with Parkinson's disease often take >5 steps
8	• Ask patient to stare at wall • Approach from above (out of sight) and repeatedly tap between their eyes	• Normally blinking stops after 2–3 taps • Look for failure of attenuation of blink response	• This is not a consistent sign • Also known as Myerson's sign
9	• Ask patient to write name/address	• Micrographia	
10	• Ask patient to undo a button	• Bradykinesia	• Patient may have Velcro in place of buttons on shirt

The Parkinson's exam: point by point in action			
	DO	**THINK!**	**EXAM TIPS**
11	• Check BP (erect and supine) • Assess eye movements • Perform cerebellar examination	• Autonomic function affected in Multiple system atrophy • Weakness of vertical gaze occurs in Progressive supranuclear palsy	• Progressive supranuclear palsy: parkinsonism associated with postural instability (falls), vertical gaze palsy, pseudobulbar palsy and dementia • Multiple system atrophy: parkinsonism associated with autonomic and cerebellar symptoms
12	• To complete my exam I would like to check the erect and supine BP (if not already done) and look at the medication chart • Thank patient	• Check for drugs used in Parkinson's disease	

Classic OSCE questions

Q1 Differential for parkinsonism

Idiopathic Parkinson's disease	
Drugs	Phenothiazine antipsychotics (e.g. chlorpromazine) GI prokinetics (e.g. metoclopramide, domperidone) Atypical antipsychotic (e.g. olanzapine), minimal risk of parkinsonism Lithium
Parkinson-plus syndrome	Multisystem atrophy Progressive supranuclear palsy
Dementia with Lewy bodies	Patients commonly have bradykinesia but less commonly tremor
Infection	HIV Syphilis
Malignancy	Frontal meningioma
Toxins	Carbon monoxide
Chronic traumatic encephalopathy (formerly dementia pugislistica)	Dementia and parkinsonism as a result of repeated head trauma (e.g. boxing)

Notes

Q2	Treatments used in Parkinson's disease
Levodopa	Most effective treatment Combined with dopa decarboxylase inhibitor to reduce peripheral side effects As disease progresses treatment becomes more difficult as patients develop on/off phenomena: • 'on' state with dopamine induced dyskinesias • 'off' state with complete immobility
Dopamine agonists	First line treatment in younger patients or used in combination with levodopa in older patients Associated with fewer motor complications than levodopa
Other drugs include:	
Selegiline	Monoamine oxidase B inhibitor Reduces catabolism of dopamine in brain
Amantadine	Increases synthesis and release of dopamine Improves dyskinesias
Antimuscarinics	Used to help tremor Adverse effects include confusion and cognitive impairment
Apomorphine	Potent dopamine agonist administered subcutaneously as a rescue during an 'off' period

Notes

Myotonic dystrophy: common OSCE openers

1. This patient presents with weakness in their limbs; please examine their muscle strength
2. This patient presents with swallowing difficulties; please examine their limbs

Myotonic dystrophy: point by point

1 Introduction (shake hands)

2 Inspection

3 Palpate facial muscles

4 Upper/lower limb tone/power

5 Tendon reflexes

6 Conclusion

Myotonic dystrophy: point by point in action

	DO	THINK!	EXAM TIPS
1	• Wash hands, introduce yourself • Confirm name/DOB	• After shaking patient's hand there will be a slow release of hand grip. This is due to continued contraction of muscles after voluntary contraction with slow, delayed relaxation (myotonia) • Speech: evidence of bulbar dysarthria?	• Look for clues at bedside, e.g. mobility aids • Myotonia can also be confirmed by asking patient to make a fist – this will be worse if cold or excited **Q1** What is the genetic basis of myotonic dystrophy?

2	• Inspect
	  • Face
	  • Chest
	  • Abdomen
	  • Limbs
		• Patient's face will have a characteristic myopathic appearance: appears sad and sleepy
		• Face: frontal baldness, ptosis, wasting of temporalis, masseters, sternocleidomastoid, neck and shoulder girdle muscles
		• Trunk: gynaecomastia, pacemaker scar (cardiac arrhythmias)
		• Abdomen: percutaneous endoscopic gastrostomy (PEG) tube present (oesophageal dysfunction)
		• Limbs: muscle wasting
			• Pupil size is normal. This helps to differentiate this condition from other causes of ptosis
			• Mild cognitive impairment may be present

Myotonic dystrophy: point by point in action			
	DO	THINK!	EXAM TIPS
3	• Palpate facial muscles	• Ask patient to open their eyes after firm closure – this will be delayed • Palpate temporalis and masseter muscles when patient clenches teeth – these will be weak	
4	• Assess tone & power in limbs	• Tone is reduced • Distal muscle weakness	• Check gait – bilateral foot drop may be present
5	• Reflexes	• Deep tendon reflexes reduced or absent	• Look for percussion myotonia – use tendon hammer to tap thenar eminence (thumb flexes)
6	• Conclude by explaining to examiner what other signs you would look for	• Eyes: cataracts • Abdomen: PEG tube (oesophageal dysfunction) • Heart: murmurs (cardiomyopathy) • Genitourinary: hypogonadism (tell examiners you could check for testicular atrophy) • Urine dip for glycosuria: diabetes mellitus is common	Q2 What further investigations would you like to perform to confirm your diagnosis?

Classic OSCE questions

Q1 What is the genetic basis of muscular dystrophy?

- Autosomal dominant
- Shows anticipation: worse symptoms in next generation
- Usually starts age 20–30 years

Q2 What further investigations would you like to perform to confirm your diagnosis?

- Genetic testing
- EMG (if genetic testing unavailable)
- Assess for associated features: blood glucose/HBA1c (diabetes mellitus), ECG (long PR, long QT, heart block), CXR (cardiomegaly, aspiration, bronchiectasis)

Note: CK will be normal

Notes

The acromegaly exam: common OSCE openers

1. This patient has noticed an increase in the size of their hands and feet; please examine them
2. This patient has noticed some changes in their vision; please examine them

The acromegaly exam: point by point

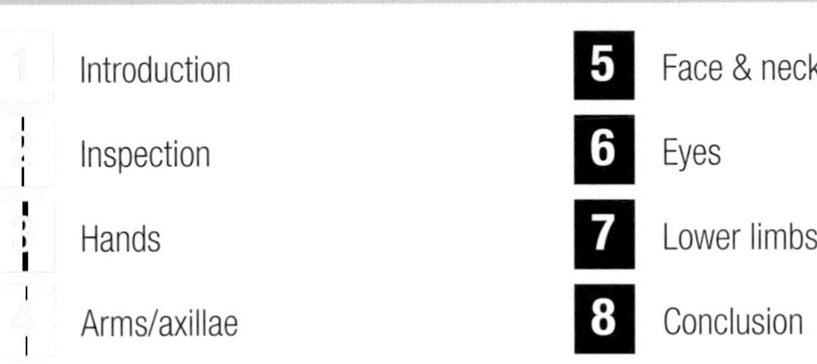

The acromegaly exam: point by point in action

	DO	THINK!	EXAM TIPS
1	• Wash hands, introduce yourself • Confirm name/DOB • Position patient at 45°	• Immediately start to assess patient's general appearance	• Features of acromegaly should be apparent from the end of the bed
2	• General inspection	• Coarse features • Thick, greasy skin	• Patients may not necessarily be tall, may be normal height with large features
3	• Inspect hands • Median nerve exam	• Wide spade-like shape • Tight fitting rings • Increased sweating in palms • Thickened skin on pinching • Thenar eminence wasting • Weakness of abduction • Sensation altered over thumb, index, middle and lateral aspect index finger • Tinel's sign and Phalen's test (see Chapter 5)	• Median nerve entrapment can occur due to carpal tunnel syndrome caused by soft tissue overgrowth
4	• Inspect arms • Check axillae	• Test power of shoulder abduction • Check axillae for skin tags	• Proximal myopathy characteristic
5	• Examine face and neck	• Prominent supraorbital ridge • Large nose, tongue • Prognathism (protrusion of mandible) • Wide separation of teeth	• As the jaw enlarges, malocclusion often develops • Patient may have a goitre (all organs may enlarge) but will be euthyroid

	The acromegaly exam: point by point in action		
	DO	**THINK!**	**EXAM TIPS**
6	• Examine eyes • Visual fields • Fundoscopy	• Assess visual fields for bitemporal hemianopia • Fundoscopy for optic atrophy (nerve compression) and papilloedema (raised intracranial pressure [ICP])	• Bitemporal hemianopia often remains after surgery • Signs of hypertensive and diabetic eye disease may be present on fundoscopy
7	• Examine lower limbs	• Ask patient to stand with arms folded (proximal myopathy) • Look for tight-fitting shoes	• Foot drop may be present due to common peroneal nerve entrapment
8	• To complete my exam I would check the blood sugar and urine for glucose. I would also check the blood pressure.	• Acromegaly commonly associated with diabetes and hypertension	

13

Confirmation of death

Common OSCE openers

You may be asked to describe how to confirm death in an OSCE station and knowing how to do this sensitively and competently is an essential prerequisite to being a doctor.

Cardiorespiratory arrest is the mode of death for the majority of patients you will see as a trainee. Death after cardiorespiratory arrest is identified by the simultaneous and irreversible onset of apnoea, unconsciousness and absence of circulation. This is what will be covered in this chapter. Secondary death of the vital centres in brainstem occurs due to the absence of circulation.

Primary brainstem death testing usually occurs in the ITU setting and is conducted by senior doctors with at least 5 years of training. This will not be covered here.

Before confirming death you must check the resuscitation status of the patient. If there is any doubt, commence CPR until this can be clarified.

Confirmation of death: point by point

1. Introduction
2. Inspection
3. Painful stimuli
4. Pupillary reflexes
5. Corneal reflexes
6. Palpate for central pulsation
7. Palpate for pacemaker
8. Auscultate for heart sounds
9. Auscultate for breath sounds
10. Update nursing staff
11. Document your findings

Confirmation of death: point by point in action

	DO	THINK!	EXAM TIPS
1	• Wash hands, introduce yourself to any family (if present) • Offer your condolences and explain what you are going to do • Offer family the opportunity to stay if they wish • Leave any bleeps with nursing staff if possible	• Ensure you have read the patient's notes in advance. Being familiar with how the patient died and whether or not this was an expected death helps you to prepare for discussions with family	• Be professional • Use your full name

2	• Confirm patient's identity (wrist band)
	• Inspect from end of bed noting colour of skin
		• Observe for:
		  • Respiratory effort
		  • Pulsations
		  • Limb movement
		• Does the patient respond to verbal stimuli?
			• Always continue to address the patient by his/her name

3	• Assess response to painful stimulus (there should be none!)	• This is best done by squeezing the trapezius muscles • Supraorbital pressure can also be used	
4	• Assess pupillary reflexes	• Shine a torchlight in each eye looking for a direct and consensual response. • Pupils should be fixed and dilated	
5	• Test for corneal reflexes with cotton wool	• Ensure the cotton wool touches the area over the iris • There should be no motor response (blinking)	• Close the eyes after examination
6	• Palpate for absence of a carotid artery pulsation	• Palpate for at least 1 minute	• This can be done at the same time as auscultation for heart sounds (point 8)
7	• Expose upper chest respectfully and palpate for a pacemaker on both sides	• Pacemakers need to be removed prior to cremation (usually done by mortuary staff)	**Q1** What is the process for signing cremation forms?
8	• Auscultate for heart sounds	• Auscultate for at least 2 minutes	• Establish that cardiorespiratory arrest has occurred for a minimum of 5 minutes
9	• Auscultate for breath sounds	• Auscultate for at least 3 minutes	

Confirmation of death: point by point in action			
	DO	**THINK!**	**EXAM TIPS**
10	• Wash hands and exit the room • Update nursing staff	• Ensure you invite the family in and explain next steps • Ensure you inform nursing staff that you have confirmed death – this will allow arrangements to be made for the patient's body to be transferred to the mortuary	**Q2** What happens after death is confirmed?
11	• Document your findings in the clinical notes	• Document each of the examination steps and the results of each step • Document date and time of death clearly • Document your name, bleep and designation clearly • If appropriate, document cause of death. This MUST be discussed with the relevant senior clinician before a death certificate can be issued • Consider whether the death needs to be referred to the Procurator Fiscal (Scotland)/ Coroner (rest of UK)	**Q3** What are the differences between Scotland and the rest of the UK with respect to the time of death? **Q4** When should you report a death to the Procurator Fiscal/ Coroner?

Classic OSCE questions

Q1 Signing cremation forms (not Scotland)

- A separate Cremation Form is required for deaths in the UK, except Scotland
- You must have seen the body after death. If you were not the doctor who confirmed death, you will need to make arrangements to inspect the body in the mortuary
- You should have treated the deceased during their last illness and have seen them within 14 days of their death

Notes

Q2 What happens after death has been confirmed?

- Relatives may want to ask questions, particularly if the death was unexpected. Familiarise yourself with the patient's history and answer any questions as accurately as you can. If you feel unable to do this, advise them that you will ask a more senior member of the team to meet with them
- Once death is confirmed, arrangements should be made to complete a death certificate (MCCD). This should be done after discussion with the patient's responsible Consultant to ensure the correct cause(s) of death are listed. Families may be asked to return to collect the certificate if there will be a delay in completing this. Ensure the death does not need to be reported to the Procurator Fiscal or Coroner **before** a certificate is issued
- Familiarise yourself with your hospital's bereavement policy. There are usually information booklets available with FAQs to support bereaved families

Q3 What are the differences between Scotland and the rest of the UK with respect to the time of death?

- In Scotland, time of death is when the patient was noted to have died, either by staff or family members
- In the rest of UK, the time of death is when death was confirmed by a doctor following the examination steps above

Notes

Q4 When should you report a death to the Procurator Fiscal/Coroner?

You should always discuss the cause of death with the patient's responsible Consultant, who can advise whether reporting to the Procurator Fiscal or Coroner is required. The table below lists the categories of deaths that should be reported. Note that this list is not exhaustive and guidance is usually available locally or by telephoning the Procurator Fiscal/Coroner's offices

Deaths that may require further investigation:

- The cause of death is unknown
- Death was violent or unnatural (includes accidents and drug related deaths)
- Death was sudden and unexplained
- The person who died was not visited by a medical practitioner during their final illness
- A medical certificate is not available
- Death occurred during an operation or before the person came round from the anaesthetic
- The medical certificate suggests that the death may have been caused by an industrial disease or industrial poisoning
- Death occurred in legal custody
- A complaint has been received over the medical treatment or standards of care received by the deceased
- Death was due to a notifiable disease
- Death of children in specific circumstances – consult your local Procurator Fiscal/Coroner guidelines

Notes

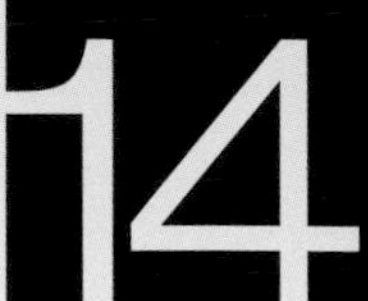

Presenting your findings

Presenting your clinical findings is a skill that you will develop with practice and experience. There are a few 'golden' rules which are outlined below and can be applied across most clinical scenarios, but most importantly it is about being confident in your own examination skills and the clinical signs you have detected.

Golden rules:

1. Stand confidently, holding your stethoscope behind your back
2. Report the positive findings of your examination
3. Do not report a list of negative findings
4. Propose a differential diagnosis consistent with your examination findings
5. Be prepared to propose an initial management plan

Below are some examples from different clinical settings of how to present your clinical findings:

Cardiovascular example

Mr. Smith is a 78-year-old gentleman who was comfortable at rest. His pulse was regular, of normal volume, and at a rate of 80 beats per minute. I felt the pulse was slow rising in character. Examination of the precordium revealed an undisplaced apex beat and on auscultation there was an ejection systolic murmur loudest in the aortic area with no radiation. The lung bases were clear and there was no evidence of ankle oedema. These findings would be consistent with a diagnosis of aortic stenosis with no signs of fluid overload. Other causes of an ejection systolic murmur include aortic sclerosis, a flow murmur and hypertrophic cardiomyopathy.

Remember:

When you are presenting, remember that the description of the murmur (e.g. ejection systolic murmur) is not the final diagnosis. You must go on to say what these findings would be consistent with (e.g. aortic stenosis) and whether there are any signs of decompensation.

Abdominal example

Mr. Smith is a 55-year-old gentleman who was comfortable at rest. He is jaundiced with finger clubbing, palmar erythema, multiple spider naevi on his trunk and gynaecomastia. He has generalised abdominal swelling with shifting dullness. His abdomen is otherwise soft and non-tender, without palpable organomegaly. He has marked peripheral oedema. The diagnosis is decompensated chronic liver disease and differentials include alcoholic liver disease, viral hepatitis, metabolic or autoimmune causes.

Remember:

The examiners may prompt you to suggest the most likely differential diagnosis, so be alert to clues which will help you narrow down the cause of chronic liver disease. Be prepared to discuss the complications of chronic liver disease.

Index

C

D

E

F

G

H

N

O

P

R

S